Women's Running **MEN'S Running**

TOTAL RUNNING

If you love to run, then *Men's Running* and *Women's Running* are the magazines for you.

THIS IS A CARLTON BOOK
Published by Carlton Books Ltd
20 Mortimer Street
London W1T 3JW

Text © Carlton Books Ltd and Wild Bunch Media Limited 2017
Design © Carlton Books 2017

ISBN 978-1-78097-992-2

Project Editor: Chris Mitchell
Design Editor: Emily Clarke and Luke Griffin
Editorial: Lucian Randall
Design: Darren Jordan
Production: Lisa Cook

A CIP catalogue for this book is available from the British Library

Printed in Dubai

10 9 8 7 6 5 4 3 2 1

Women's Running **MEN'S Running**

TOTAL RUNNING

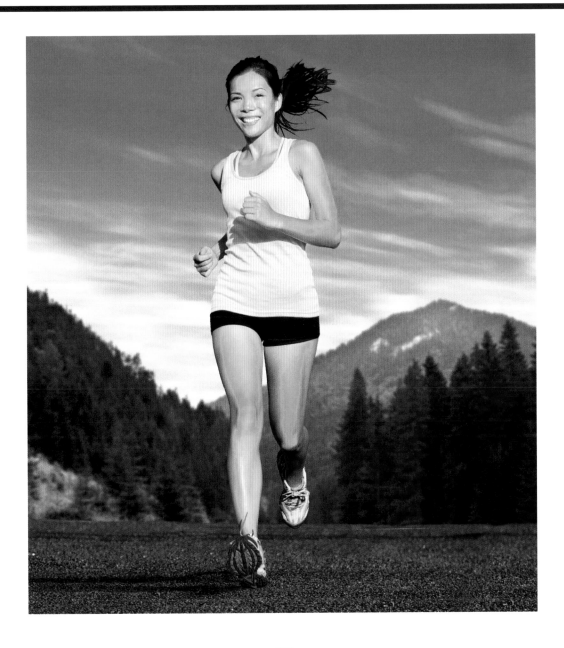

CARLTON
BOOKS

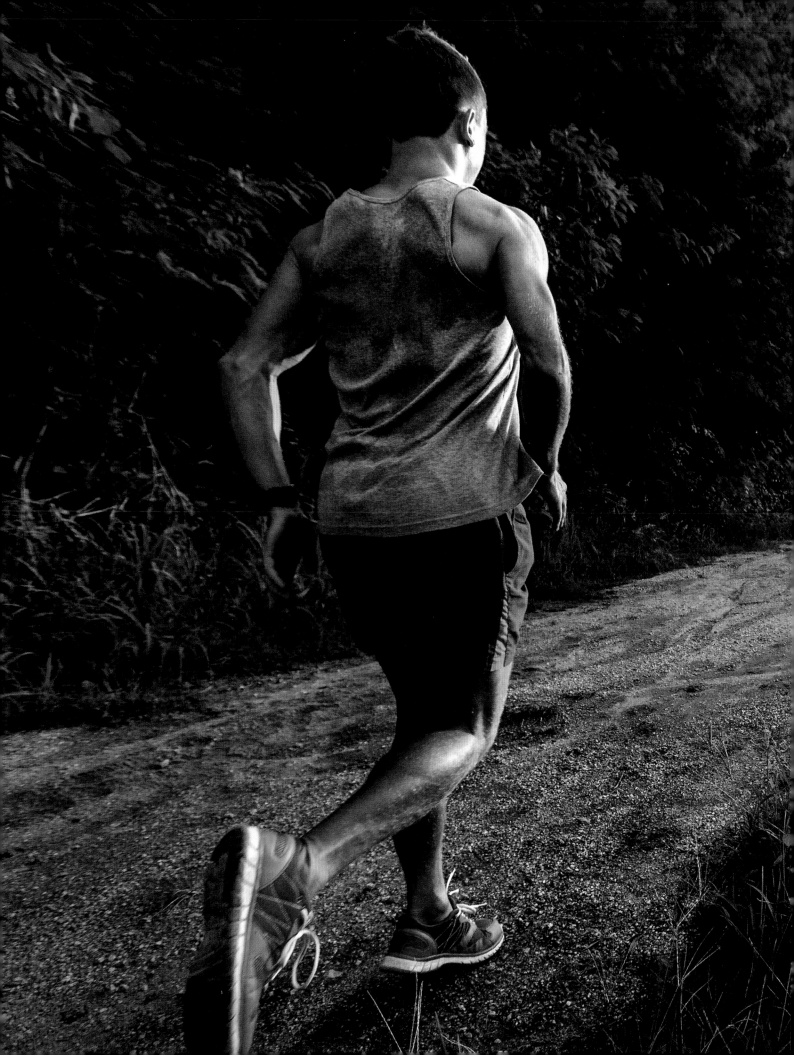

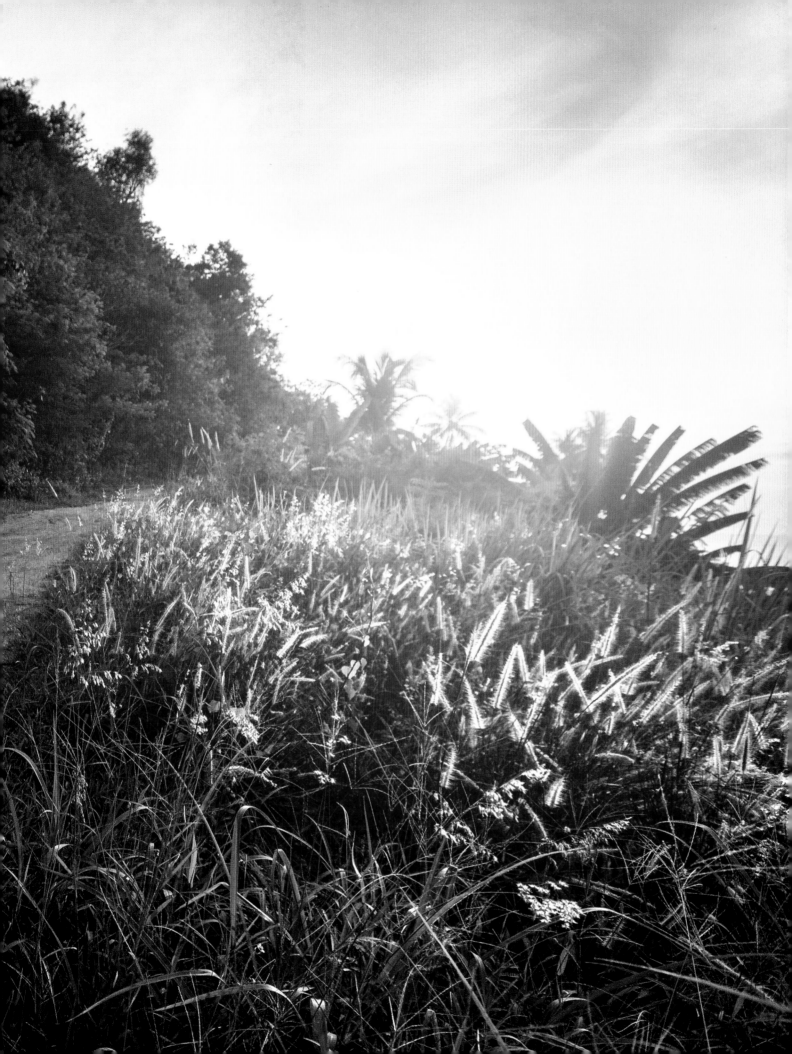

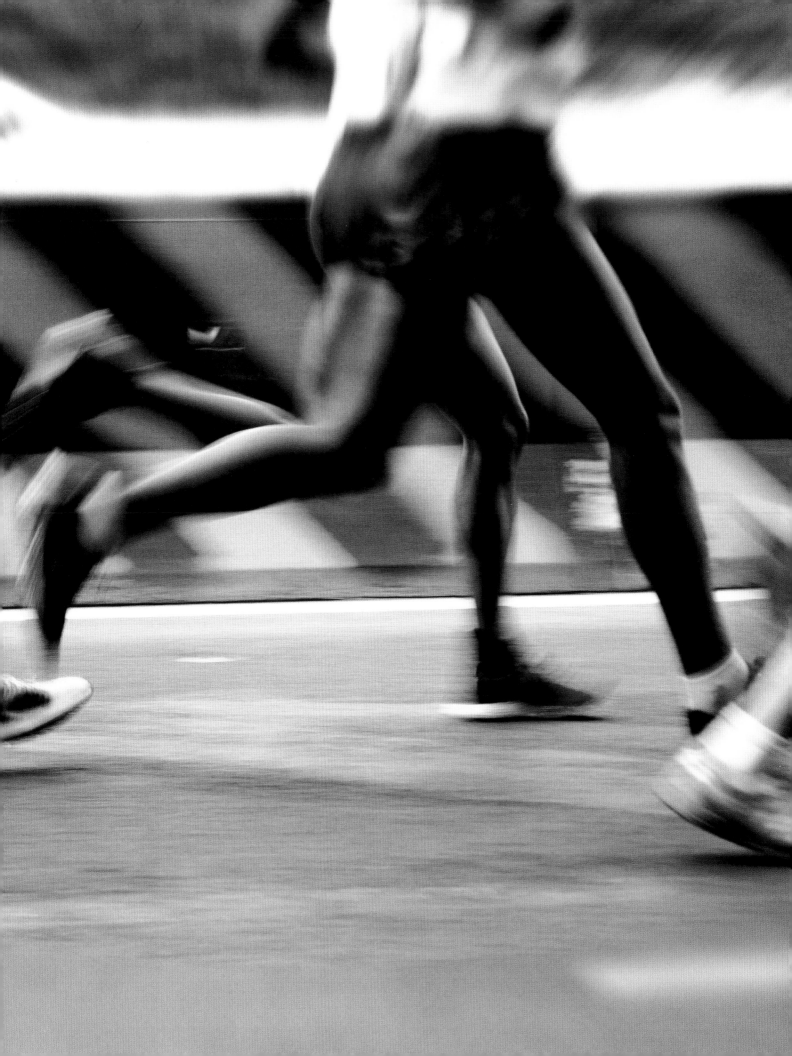

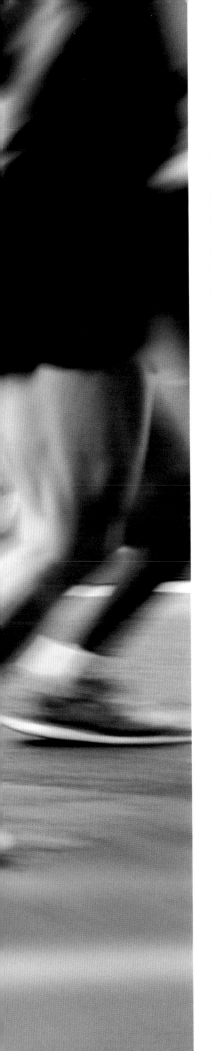

CONTENTS

INTRODUCTION

"Do you remember your first run?" It's a question I get asked all the time. The reality is I don't. But even though I've been running for longer than I can remember (or would be prepared to admit to!), I still get the same feelings that I would have done all those years ago - the sense of freedom, that ability to be at one with the world, to leave the real world behind and focus on the simple act of putting one foot in front of the other.

That's the beauty of running: it really is the simplest of sports and, pound-for-pound, one of the best ways to get fit. All you need is a decent pair of trainers, some basic kit and off you go. Of course, if you're reading this book, then you will have already taken the decision to start your own running journey. Congratulations! Designed for beginners and improvers alike, this book contains everything you need to help you get your shoes on and out the door.

Everyone has a different entry point into the sport. You could be running for weight loss or to get fit; you could have been inspired by a big race; or you could be running to raise funds in memory of a loved one. Whatever your

rationale, this book will be a vital component of your running journey, a coach, a friend and companion to help you reach whatever goal you have in mind.

For me, running has been a key decision maker in my life. Influencing the choice of university I went to and to go on to become a journalist and working for a running magazine, running has afforded me opportunities I would have never experienced. From climbing the highest mountain in Mauritius to running the cobbles in Rome; from running the Bob Marley mile in Jamaica to running a sub 5-minute mile in a car park under Marble Arch, running has been the one constant in my life.

For anyone taking their first steps into running, or looking to improve on the ones they have already taken, this book is an essential read. If you're looking for inspiration to run, advice on how and what to do and a guide to all things running, then read on. I hope that you will be as inspired in your own running journeys as I have. And that you, of course, always remember that first run!

David Castle
Editorial Director, Wild Bunch Media

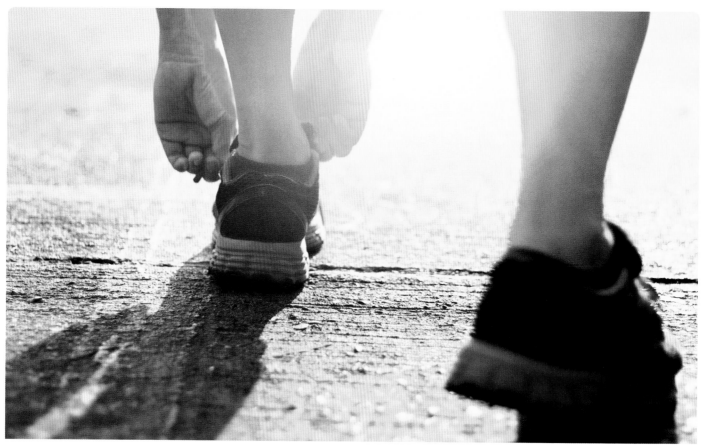

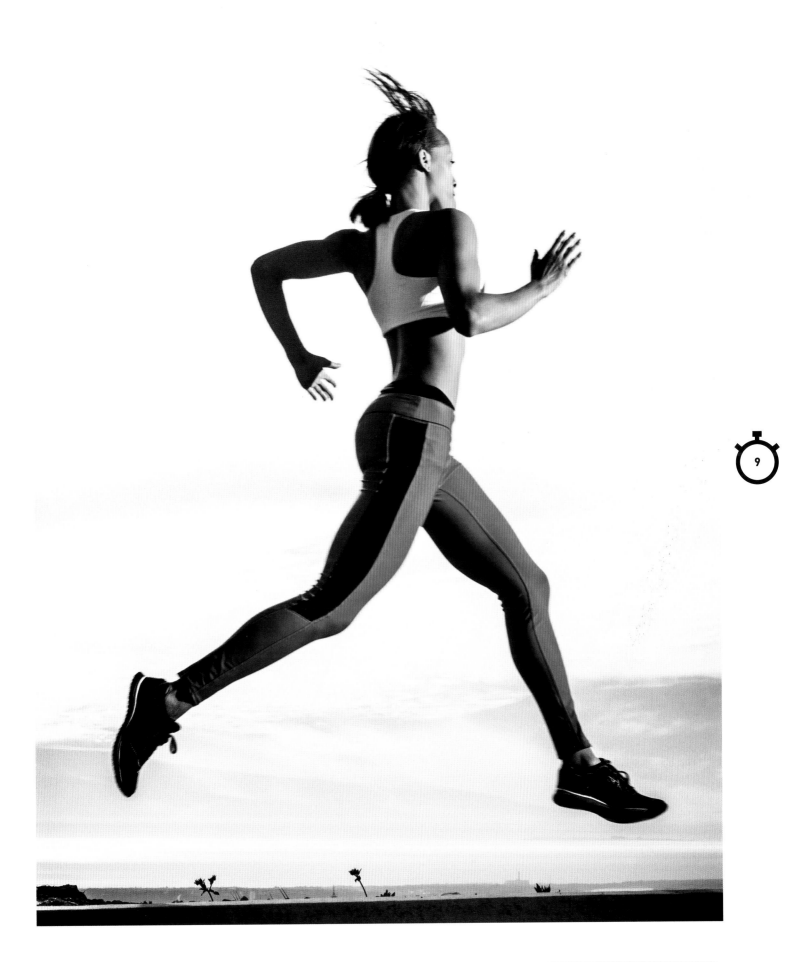

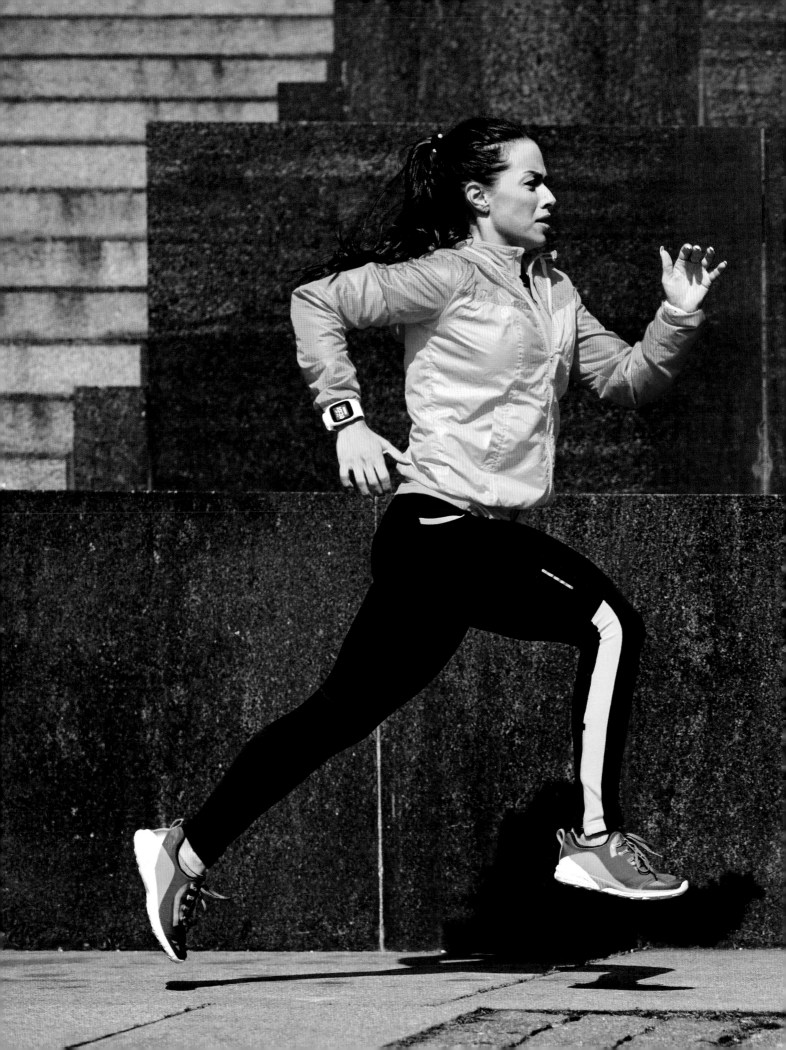

GETTING STARTED

All you need to get you out of the door and onto the pavement, into the park or out on the trails. It's surprisingly easy to get started in running and find out how to get a decent pair of shoes. It helps to know what you want to achieve, but otherwise you can be out there running almost immediately.

REASONS TO RUN

Experts say that regular running provides many health benefits and can prolong your life. Even if you're unfit or overweight that doesn't need to stop you.

RUN FOR YOUR LIFE

Regular running can help you live longer, even if you're only jogging or covering short distances. Heart expert Dr Peter Schnoh, who led a study of 2,000 male and female joggers, looked at death rates of more than 1,100 males and more than 760 females over a 35-year timeframe. The data showed that jogging increased the lifespan of men by 6.2 years and women by 5.6 years. Compared with non-runners, the risk of death for both sexes was reduced by 44 per cent.

PHYSICAL HEALTH BENEFITS

12

A study undertaken at Stanford University looked at runners' heart health over 20 years and found that older runners were at less risk of heart disease than their peers. Cancer Research UK says that regular exercise like running can reduce bowel cancer risk by increasing the rate at which food moves through the bowels, reducing the amount of time the lining of the bowel is in contact with harmful chemicals released through consumption of red meat or alcohol. Running can also reduce risk of stroke by 20 to 40 per cent, type 2 diabetes and breast cancer risk in women both by 30 per cent, as well as reducing dementia risk by 30 per cent. So the message is clear – want to live longer? Start running!

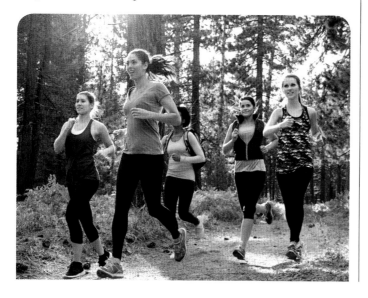

YOUR HEALTH QUESTIONS ANSWERED

It's best to get the all-clear from your GP first and then build up distance and volume gradually. Start with short runs – five to ten minutes will be fine – and you can walk/run too. "If you are unfit, start by including small bursts of exercise in your day, such as walking at a moderate to fast pace to the next bus stop or taking the stairs at work," says Dr Tatiana Lapa, a GP and medical director of The Studio.

CAN RUNNING BRING ON A HEART ATTACK IF I HAVE HIGH CHOLESTEROL OR HIGH BLOOD PRESSURE?

"Have a regular check-up with your doctor at least once a year, especially if you are about to start on a new exercise programme," says Lapa. "Having dangerously high blood pressure levels puts you at risk of having serious health problems such as heart attack or stroke." Dangerously high means a systolic reading (when the heart contracts)

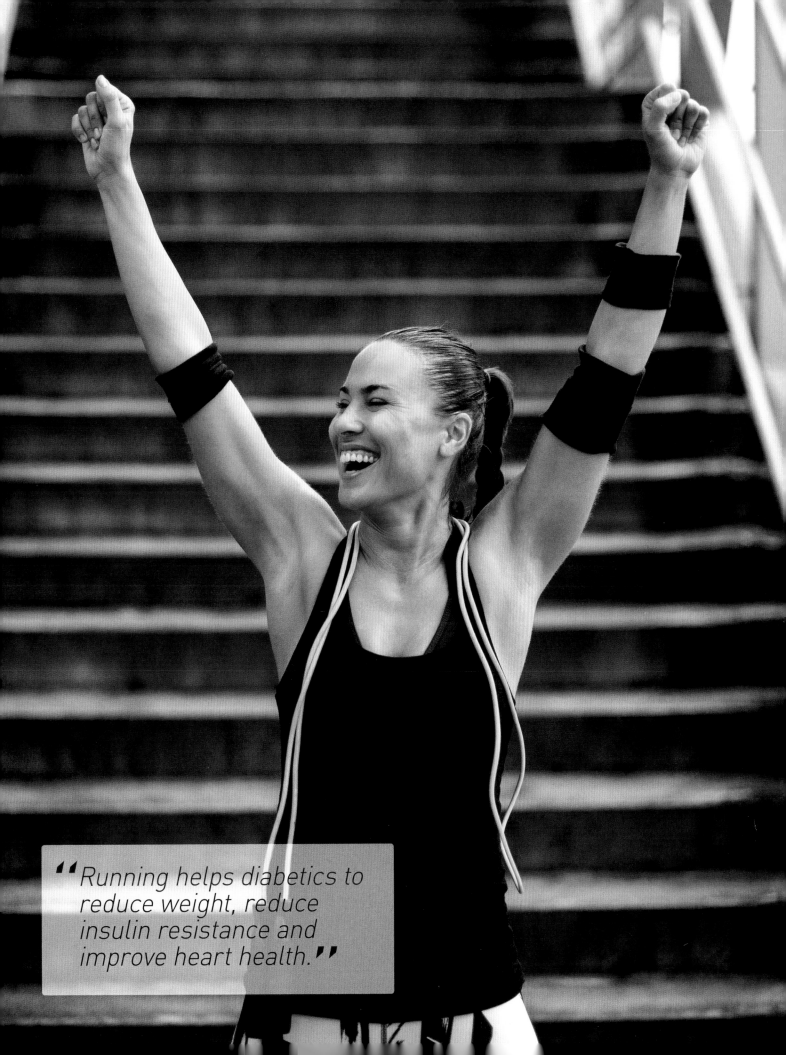

> "Running helps diabetics to reduce weight, reduce insulin resistance and improve heart health."

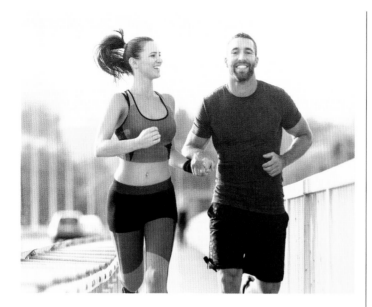

CAN I RUN IF I'M OVERWEIGHT?

"Yes, it's a great thing to do if you're overweight and you'll soon see the benefits as it will help you lose weight," says Kipps. "Build up slowly, don't go too far or too fast too soon, as you'll risk injury."

WILL RUNNING WITH ARTHRITIS MAKE IT WORSE OR CAUSE KNEE PROBLEMS IN LATER LIFE?

"The evidence shows that the risk of osteoarthritis is no more in runners than sedentary individuals – provided they have no previous injuries," says Kipps. "The key is to build up slowly and not over-exert too soon. It also helps to do some strengthening exercises for the back, hips and core to optimise control and develop technique for reducing the chance of developing other injuries. Seek professional advice."

EMOTIONAL BENEFITS

It has long been known that running can improve mood and help us to cope with stress. We can even use it to help manage our emotions. A run can clear our heads and make us feel better, even in extreme situations such as bereavement. "If something traumatic has happened, going for a run can be a really good opportunity to break things down," says Philip Clarke, a psychology lecturer at the University of Derby. "A run can be a really good opportunity to make sense of situations in your head. It also means you may run further. If you're focusing on a situation, it can take away the feeling of perceived exertion. First of all, any exercise releases endorphins. You feel a lot happier for it. At the end of the day, it's a happy drug."

IN CONTROL

For many of us, running can give us back a much-needed sense of control to help us manage stress. "A lot of emotions come from uncontrollable things like stress at work, relationships and family illness," says Clarke. "You often have no control over some of those things, whereas your body and your running can be a real source of control because you're in charge. It's up to you whether you go out and do 5K or 10K or if you stop. That's something you have complete control over and that's why people use it."

But can running help us make sense of our problems? "There is a fantastic quote from an ancient philosopher, Lao-Tse, which beautifully captures the potential of exercise in helping to overcome life's difficulties," says Dr Tracey Devonport, a sport and exercise psychologist at the University of Wolverhampton. "'It is as though she/he listened and such listening enfolds us in a silence in which, at last, we begin to hear what we are meant to be'. Exercising on our own provides us with space to think and to process what is going on in our lives. Or if we run with others, they can be our sounding board, to simply listen, perhaps offer advice or a different perspective."

of 180 or higher or a diastolic reading (when the heart relaxes) of 110 or higher, so having high blood pressure under this range shouldn't stop you from exercising and it should benefit your health, provided you've had the all-clear from your GP. "Those with a family history of heart disease need to clarify the exact type of heart disease," says Lapa, so make sure you consult your GP.

"Running is a positive step," says Dr Courtney Kipps, sports and exercise specialist at the UK's Institute of Sports Exercise and Health. "Exercise will reduce risk, not increase it."

14

CAN I RUN IF I'VE BEEN DIAGNOSED WITH TYPE 2 DIABETES?

"Exercise such as running is very important in the management of type 2 diabetes," says Lapa. "Running helps diabetics to reduce weight, reduce insulin resistance and improve heart health. Type 2 diabetes is often a progressive condition, with the majority of people needing to use insulin within ten years of diagnosis. Exercise and weight loss can slow this progression down and, in some cases, can even help type 2 diabetics revert back to normal health."

Caution is needed though, as some treatments for diabetes can cause blood sugar levels to drop, resulting in hypoglycaemia (low blood glucose). "Exercise can also cause blood sugar levels to drop," says Lapa. "Diabetics using insulin should be aware of signs of hypoglycaemia, check their sugar levels prior to starting exercise and at 30-minute intervals during exercise."

If your blood sugar level is below 7 mmol/L, the Association of British Clinical Diabetologists recommends consuming 30 g of carbohydrate before exercise.

Is it safe to run with asthma?

"It is safe for well-controlled asthmatics to exercise," says Lapa. "If [your] asthma is made worse by exercise, then see your GP or asthma nurse. Some asthma symptoms may be triggered by pollen allergies, so it may be useful to use antihistamines or nasal spray. Have your reliever inhaler on hand in case of worsening symptoms."

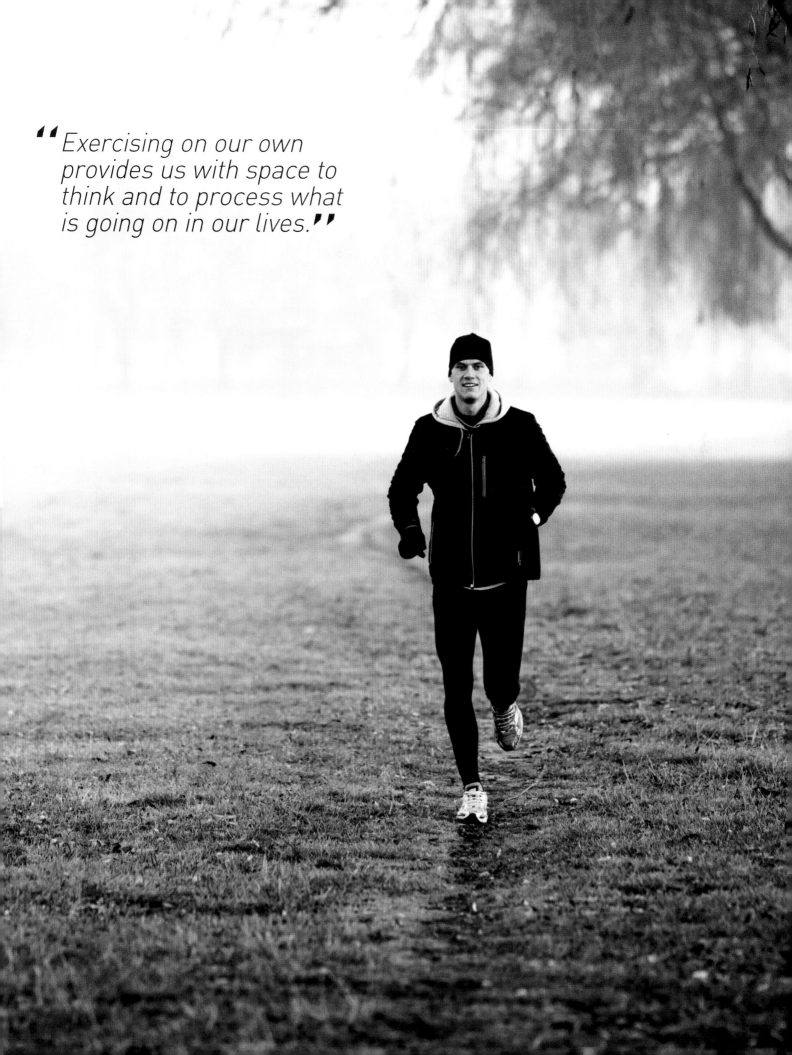

"Exercising on our own provides us with space to think and to process what is going on in our lives."

THE TEN COMMANDMENTS FOR NEW RUNNERS

Live by these ten principles and you won't go far wrong.

1 IT'S A MARATHON NOT A SPRINT
As a beginner, it's important to remember that, no matter how little you currently run, or how big your running ambitions might be, the best way to succeed is to follow a steady and progressive plan. Allow yourself time to build up distance and speed gradually and you'll enjoy a long and successful running career. Pile on the miles too fast and you'll end up injured and waste days or weeks recovering and feeling fed up.

2 LEARN TO LISTEN TO YOUR BODY
To make life easy, use training schedules (see Chapter 6) to fast-track your progress towards great results. Remember, however, that feedback from your body will always be the most important indicator of how hard you push yourself. If you experience any aches, pains, fatigue or unexpected tiredness, take time to rest and recover, regardless of what your training plan says. Only add training to a healthy and well-prepared body and mind; don't expect much response if you start a training session feeling weak, wobbly and exhausted.

3 DEVELOP A SUPPORT TEAM
Be proactive with how you maintain your best running fitness by regularly checking in with your 'team' of specialists. The occasional appointment with a physiotherapist, podiatrist, chiropractor or massage therapist can keep you in tip-top shape and greatly reduce the chance of developing any injuries.

4 VARIETY IS THE SPICE OF RUNNING
The greater the variety in your training terrain, the quicker your fitness gains will be. Running up and downhill will improve basic speed and the strength in your legs so make sure you regularly incorporate hill runs of varying distances and inclines. Include sprint training as well whether this be running chosen sections of some routes faster or by visiting a running track for some all-out efforts.

5 RUNNING IS NOT JUST ABOUT RUNNING
Balance the physical motion of running by including regular strength training, core work and flexibility training.

Also consider elements of yoga, Pilates or cross-training such as cycling, swimming, rowing or circuit training.

6 CHALLENGE YOURSELF
Test your abilities against the clock or other runners. Racing or signing up for charity events are great ways of structuring your training schedule and pushing yourself a little bit harder.

7 TRAIN WITH A PARTNER OR JOIN A CLUB
Whether it be with a friend, training partner or members of a running club, regular interaction with other runners will keep you motivated and help you uncover new training ideas.

8 KEEP YOURSELF REGULAR
Don't worry about missing a run if you need to recover or you're following a scheduled break, but do aim to keep your running routine as regular as possible. Irregular or sporadic training leaves you feeling as though you're often playing catch-up having made progress. If you're pushed for time you can make training runs as short as five minutes and they'll still count. Time pressure makes you creative with your training plans. Even two or three minutes can make a massive difference to how you feel physically and mentally.

9 RUNNING MAKES THE WORLD A BRIGHTER PLACE
Even on the gloomiest of days you'll feel better after a run. Run to beat a previous time, run to help you wake up, run to solve a work problem or run to blow out some stress. Make the effort to get out there – you won't regret it.

10 THE RIGHT KIT IS ESSENTIAL
Kitting yourself out with appropriate trainers, clothing and technology really can make the difference between an average running career and one that quickly goes from strength to strength (see pp.24–31). Get comfortable, wear clothing that's appropriate to the conditions you're training in and use technology to track your progress and fine-tune your training schedule. Above all, get yourself to a specialist running store to make sure you have the right shoes on your feet and reduce your chance of injury.

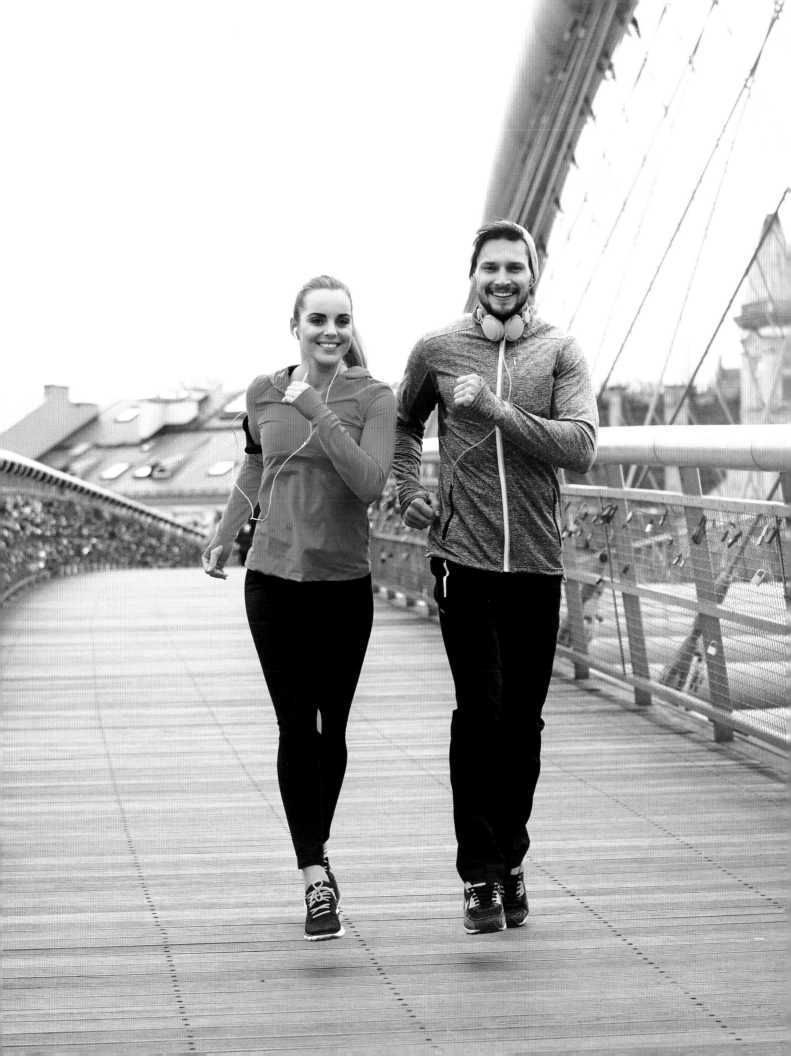

THE BASICS

It isn't hard to make a good start with your new passion, to run well and reduce the risk of injury.

The great thing about running is that it's straightforward. You just pull on your trainers and you can get going at a moment's notice. As you become a regular runner, there are a number of things you'll learn that make running easier. This is information that many runners only discover through painful experience and this is how you will save unnecessary time and effort.

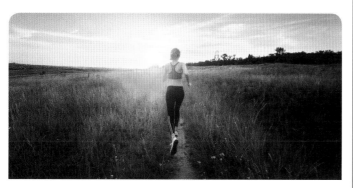

START SLOWLY AND BUILD UP

Increasing mileage too quickly doesn't allow your body time to adapt to the demands being made on it and the result is that you could risk injury. Building your weekly distances up gradually will ensure your fitness improves progressively and consistently. Set yourself some benchmarks and objectives. Measure your speed, times and distance regularly and watch your progress improving. It can be extremely satisfying.

Don't settle for always running at a consistent, steady speed. Once you've made that commitment to get out there and run on a regular basis, mix up your training with some hill running, intervals and speed work, to maximise your fitness gains.

FUEL YOURSELF PROPERLY

It's important to make nutrition a key foundation stone of your running. There will be more detail on that in the chapter beginning on p.126. But in general, you need to being thinking about it all the time; not just before and after your runs, but throughout each day, every day. 'Fuelling' your body regularly with the right food and drink will help you burn calories more efficiently when you run and this will improve your stamina. Good fuelling will also help you with your recovery between runs.

TIP

If you experience blisters, simply pierce a hole at the edge of the blister and squeeze out any liquid. Leave the skin on the blister and apply Vaseline.

Hydrate yourself regularly throughout each day. Don't drink too much water prior to a run and don't hit the pavements dehydrated. Get into the routine of sipping water or an energy drink or gel as you run and tune into your running-related toilet routine. For those longer runs, you should know how far you can run before you'll need to go to the loo so you can plan toilet breaks on the way.

STRETCH AFTER EACH RUN

Not only is stretching important (see pp.98–101), you should also spend 10 to 20 minutes at least once a week devoted only to stretching. This may not feel as though it's getting you fitter or helping with your running, but over the course of weeks, months and years, these stretching sessions could be the vital ingredient in your training routine that keeps you on the road.

TRAIN EVERY TWO OR THREE DAYS

Working out frequently is enough to ensure quick progress with your fitness, while allowing you sufficient rest and recovery, which is vital as this is the time when your body becomes stronger and fitter. This pattern is also easier to manage psychologically. Aiming to work out too frequently can be difficult to accommodate and will leave you frustrated if it doesn't happen. At the same time, if you have any nagging doubts that you are less than a hundred per cent or feel there's a reason why you shouldn't run today, pay attention to those feelings. Better to wait a day and be fully fit, focused and looking forward to your exercise than to drag yourself out half-heartedly. A lack of focus when you're running is more likely to put you at risk of accident or injury.

And, finally – breathe! When you run, focus your breathing deep into your lungs. Oxygen transfer is more efficient when you breathe deeply, so it will make your running feel noticeably easier.

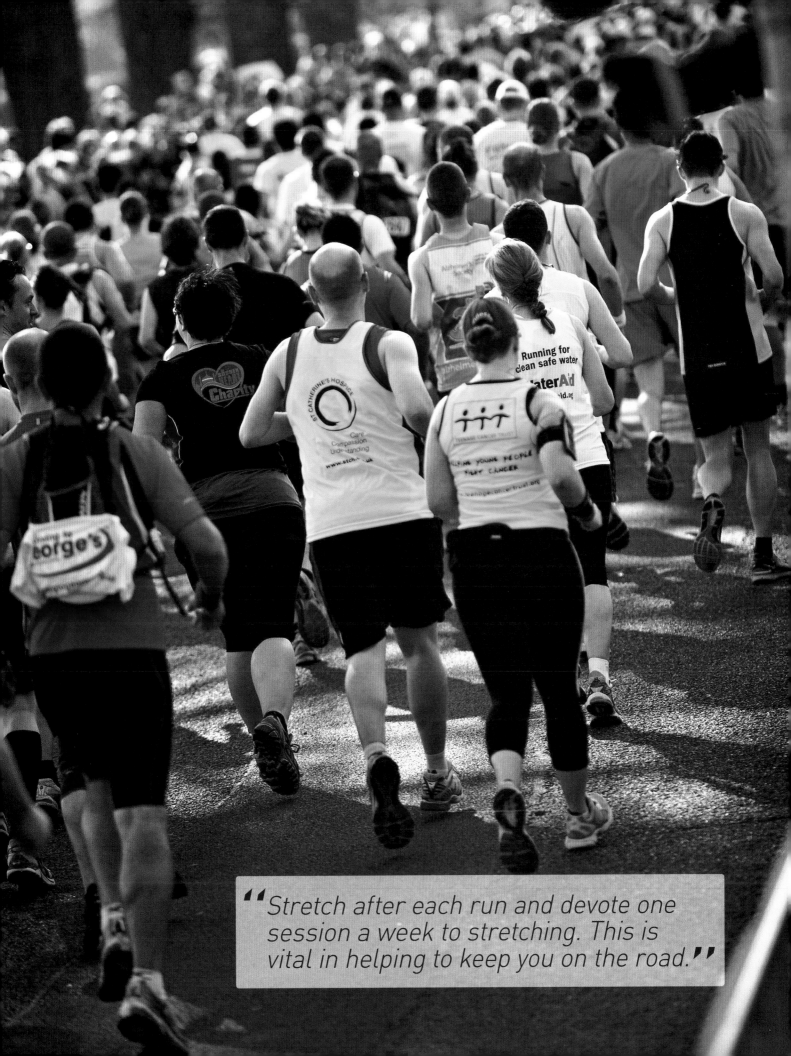

"Stretch after each run and devote one session a week to stretching. This is vital in helping to keep you on the road."

STAYING SAFE

It's all very well starting your running career in the summer, but you want to keep going all year round, when it gets colder and darker. Make sure you are good to go whatever the weather.

As winter draws on, colder, darker evenings change the landscape of many of your runs. Whether you run on your own or in a group, suddenly every kerb can be a hazard and any stretch of your unlit route is potentially dangerous.

There are some basic rules you can follow to try to ensure your own safety in the dark. If you can always stick to lit areas for nighttime runs it's obvious you'll feel safer. In built up areas it's also important you stay highly visible, even when running with friends. Wearing a reflective vest or a light during winter sessions means that you are visible to approaching cars. Headlights bounce light back off reflective material.

There are many different grades of reflective material. Some are cheaper and may not last as long, whereas others will meet certified reflective standards – these are the best pieces of kit to invest in. Reflective piping on clothing that runs down the seams is generally good quality and is integrated in to the garment itself so it won't peel. The best products you can buy are those either made completely out of reflective material, or have large patches of reflective material. This is not stuck on, but rather the material forms part of the garment.

It may be worth investing in good quality winter kit to ensure you are as bright as you can be. Various reflective materials may look similar in the daylight (silver in colour), but not all silver is created equally. Reflective brightness (RA) is the measurement scale and 100 RA is the minimum light required in many occupational settings. It's a good guide to help you make your choice at the checkout. Make sure as much of you is covered as possible, particularly motion points such as your wrists and ankles.

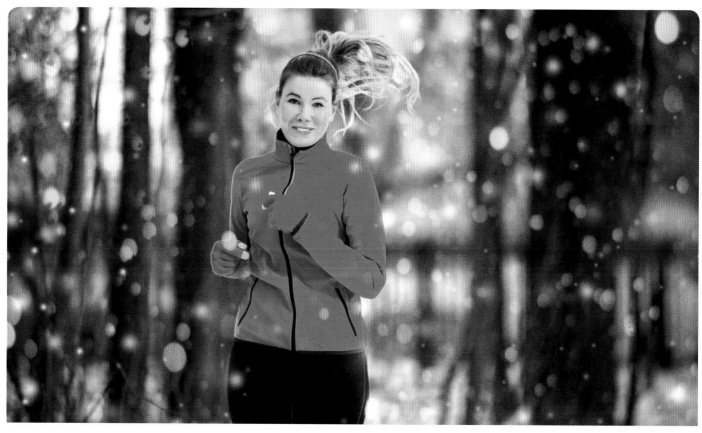

GET YOUR KIT ON

Fluorescent kit will also help keep you visible, especially during gloomy days, but at night, early in the morning, or during any other low-light times and environments, it's important to wear reflective material as well: combining both in your chosen clothes is the perfect solution.

"*Above all, trust your instincts.***"**

BE BRIGHT ABOUT THE DARK

There's no reason why you should shy away from running in the dark. Be sensible and get the right kit.

• Plan your route in advance and avoid less populated and unlit/poorly lit areas

• If you are running alone then tell someone where you are going to run and what time they should expect you back

• If you are running on the pavement, ensure you run on the side of the road that puts you facing oncoming traffic

• Vary your running route and/or the time of the day you go out

• Avoid wearing headphones when you are out, as they prevent you from hearing danger approaching

• Carry a personal alarm with you as this can be used to disorientate a potential attacker

• Carry a mobile phone and a small amount of money out of sight in case of emergency

• Wear high visibility and reflective clothing

• Avoid pushing yourself to your absolute limit so that you have the energy to run away if you are in a dangerous situation

• Above all, trust your instincts

21

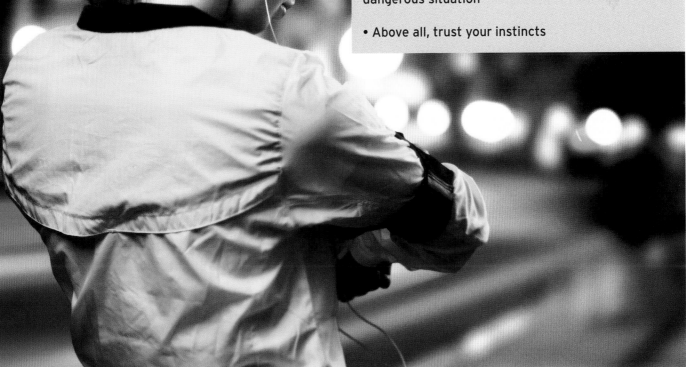

HOW TO RUN YOUR FIRST 10K

Even if you're only putting your trainers on for the first time, there's no reason not to aim for completing your first 10K.

It can seem like a daunting challenge – 10K (ten kilometres is the equivalent of a six-mile race). But even if you're a complete newbie, you can set 10K as a doable challenge. There are plenty of races out there to choose from and there may well be one near you. It's all about the training to add distance.

plans in Chapter 6 for more ideas.

When you first start to run, you can quickly become out of breath, which can feel scary if you haven't done this since school. But it is normal. It's definitely something to avoid in a race, when the biggest mistake for new runners is going off too fast. How do you know you have done this?

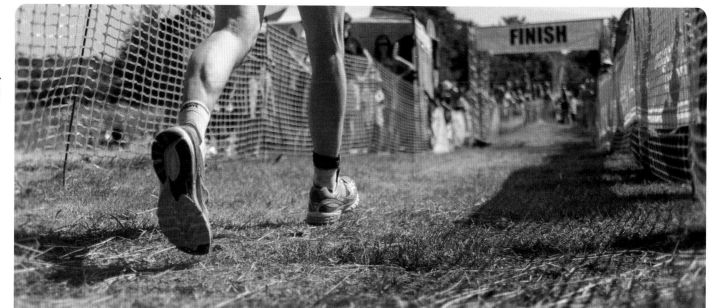

Training for a 10K is similar to a 5K, however the distance of your long runs will double. A common misconception is that you need to have run the distance in training before race day: you don't. If you've run five miles, the occasion will pull you through the last mile.

DON'T OVERDO IT

There are three key weekly sessions – a long run, a 30-minute steady run and an interval session. Interval running is about running faster over a short distance, then recovering before you repeat the effort. This helps your body get used to the feeling of running fast, and helps your heart and lungs adapt to let you do this. Take a look at our training

Think of the perceived effort you are running at on a scale of 1–10. One is walking, ten is running as fast as you can. If you are at 8–10, it's too fast! You should be aiming for 6–7 to be able to finish comfortably. If you're too fast to begin with, don't panic. Break the remaining distance down into periods of running, then walking for two minutes to recover, before trying to run again for two minutes.

Nail your pacing on race day by monitoring your breathing and ability to talk while moving. For a first 10K, it's unlikely that you are chasing a time, so you won't be running flat out. Aim to be able to speak 8–10 words with the person next to you before you have to take a breath and before you know it that finish line will appear.

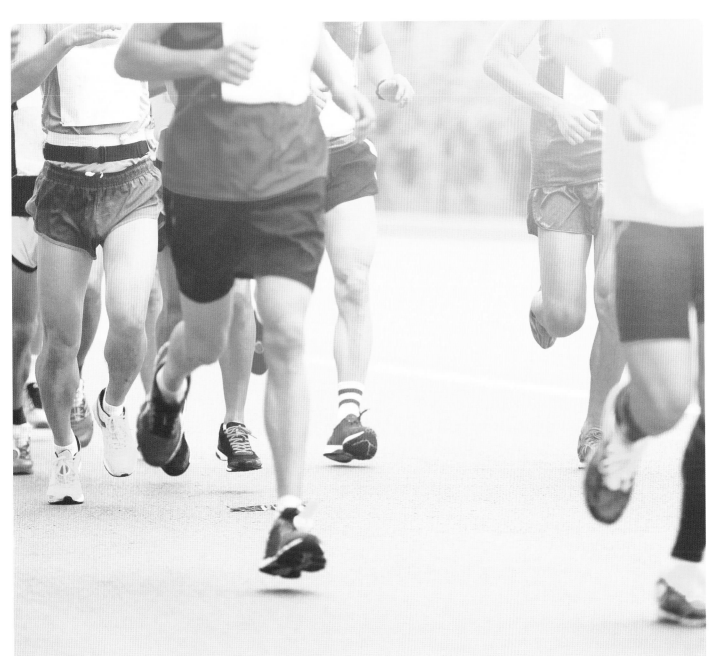

BALANCE YOUR DIET

A body loaded with junk is too busy detoxifying to thrive, leading to fatigue, low energy levels and faster burnout when it comes to race day. Try cooking with grains that have a low glycaemic index and aren't processed, such as amaranth and quinoa. Processed, refined sugary foods such as white bread and pasta don't offer much nutritionally other than carbohydrate and "empty" calories. Healthy fats, such as free-range eggs and organic avocados, quality proteins such as sustainable, organic chicken and fish such as salmon are important, as are seasonal fruits, vegetables and spices. These are anti-inflammatory and are rich in antioxidants, aiding the recovery process. Seek out iron-rich foods, including dark-green leafy vegetables such as kale, spinach, broccoli and dark-coloured berries.

Eat your pre-race breakfast two to three hours before your run to allow the food to be digested. It's also important to refuel and rehydrate as quickly as possible after running in order to reduce muscle soreness and boost energy levels.

MOTIVATION IS KEY

You need to find out the core 'why' or motivation for running: the bottom-line reason behind your effort. For example, if you are running with a friend, ask yourself why? If it's to support them as they raise money for charity, why do you want to help? Keep going until there are no more questions – this is your core motivation. When those last-minute nerves kick in, don't let them stop you achieving success. Connect with others for external energy to boost your confidence or look inside yourself. You can do it!

LET YOUR SHOES SHINE

You're going to be wearing your running shoes for a long time so make sure you get the right pair.

It should go without saying that if you are going to pound the road for any distance you need to be confident you are giving your feet the tools they need to perform. Choosing a perfect race shoe is a personal business (one runner's well-cushioned shoe is another's pointless weight) but here are some key points to consider when you're trying to choose from the massive range of shoes out there.

YOU'VE GOT TO ROLL WITH IT

Knowing how your body moves and how your foot strikes the ground when you run should be central when buying race shoes. Whether you heel-strike, midfoot- or forefoot-strike, whether you have neutral gait or whether you pronate (roll inwards) or supinate (strike on the outside of your foot) will affect the amount of cushion or support you require and feel comfortable with.

Go to a good running shop and ask for your gait to be analysed before you buy your shoes. You might be surprised at the level of experience and expertise on offer – many running stores are staffed by club runners who can help you understand what you need.

HOW LONG TO KEEP YOUR SHOES

It isn't always easy to know when to buy new running shoes. If you wait until you can feel the tarmac on the soles of your feet, the chances are you have been risking injury for hundreds of miles. The cushioning in your shoes loses its effectiveness some time before the soles wear out enough for you to notice. If you keep training plans and logs, note when you have put in 4-500 miles in the same pair of shoes. That's when it's time to retire them.

IF THE SHOE FITS

Everyone likes a shoe that fits, well, like a glove, but be aware that your feet will swell when you do high mileages, increasing your chances of blisters and cramping if they have no space in which to expand. Shop for your shoes after a short run or at the end of the day, when your feet have swollen through the course of the day. Wear whatever you would usually have as running socks and give yourself about 0.5-1 cm space between the tip of your big toe and the end of the shoe. Consider replacing the laces with elasticated laces, which keep your feet snug while allowing the upper of your shoes to expand as your feel swell.

MINIMALISM

The degree of support and cushioning you need for short runs will be different to that needed when you get up to marathon distances. There is a huge range of shoes on the market to cater for every occasion, from racing flats to heavily

24

> *"Shop for your shoes after a short run or at the end of the day."*

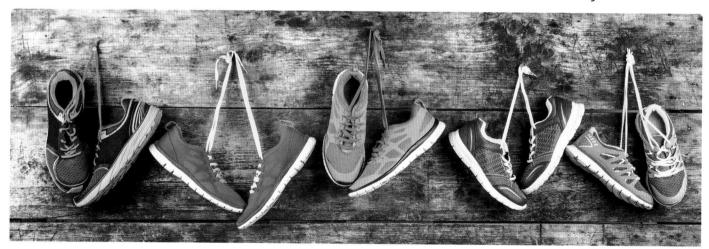

cushioned, rubber bricks. Flatter, more minimalist shoes can be attractive for racing, but a lower profile shoe can also put more strain on your Achilles tendons and calf muscles.

If you do get into racing, a relatively light shoe can be an advantage in some respects but don't compromise on support and cushioning. Always give yourself time to adapt before trying to race in new shoes. If in doubt, go for extra comfort, cushioning and support. Forget cool brands or good looks – it's all about the fit. Never buy new kit near to a race or, worse yet, on the day! You always need to gradually break in new shoes and allow the cushioning and uppers to relax before you are ready to race in them. Give yourself enough time to run a good number of miles in your shoes before you try to race in them. Wear them on a long run and during a couple of your race-pace sessions. Then they'll be ready for race day and so will you.

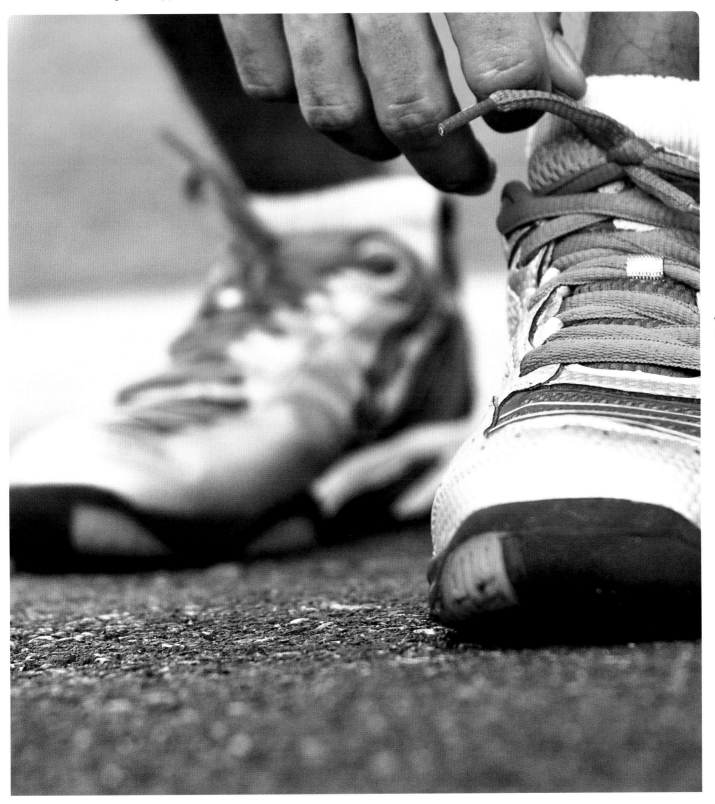

ALL THE KIT

You don't need to invest a fortune to have a diverse running wardrobe for all occasions.

As long as you have very good shoes (see pp.24-5), you can take your time in stocking up on the rest of your gear. You may have started off on a treadmill indoors and are only now contemplating stepping outside to vary your running. But don't worry about those cold days – according to running experts (and runners!), there's no such thing as it being too cold to run, but there is such a thing as wearing the wrong clothing on a run.

By investing in a few essentials you van be sure you don't get too cold or hot to run comfortably. Whatever the temperature outside, you can be sure that you'll be warm or cool enough and generally comfortable during all runs.

BE SEEN

If you're going to be running on dark early mornings or evenings, some form of reflective high-visibility kit is essential so that car drivers, cyclists and other pedestrians can see you. If you don't like the idea of buying a high-visibility orange or yellow jacket, invest in a high-vis top or at least make sure that some of your clothing has reflective strips so that you can definitely be seen. It's not unusual for cars to hit runners who don't stand out in badly lit areas, so don't risk your safety. If you're not a big fan of running jackets, you can buy high-vis long- sleeved running tops. You can also buy water-repellent and high-vis jackets, so you won't need to invest in a separate waterproof jacket and you can be assured of being seen at all times. A baseball cap will help keep the rain out of your eyes and there are many caps with high-vis strips that help keep you safe.

RACE-DAY KIT CHECKLIST

Don't leave home without these items...

• Running shoes - make sure they are broken in; never wear new shoes. And take spare laces.

• Running shorts, leggings, socks and running top - if all your gear is new, ensure you have washed it before you race in it. Feeling as if you have worn it will make you feel more prepared.

• Sports bra - take a spare one, just in case.

• Waist belt - you'll need this to store energy gels, change and a mobile phone during the race.

• A waterproof jacket - have this to keep warm before the race and to put on afterwards as you will cool down quickly once you finish

• Bin bag or old spare top - it's essential to keep warm on race morning once you've dropped off your kit bag.

• Mobile phone - to meet up with friends and family.

Keep it switched off during the run to save battery.

• Vaseline - a must if you want to avoid chafing. And you do!

• Plasters - a small first-aid kit is a must.

• Snack foods - such as bananas, muesli bars, chocolate and energy gels.

• Water and energy drinks - you never know when you might need them.

• Safety pins - to attach your race number to your top.

• Race number, information and course map - read and reread the information that the organisers send. You can never know too much!

• GPS watch - and remember to hand your chip in at the end of the race, so you can get your official time.

• Cash - for emergency purchases before or after the race.

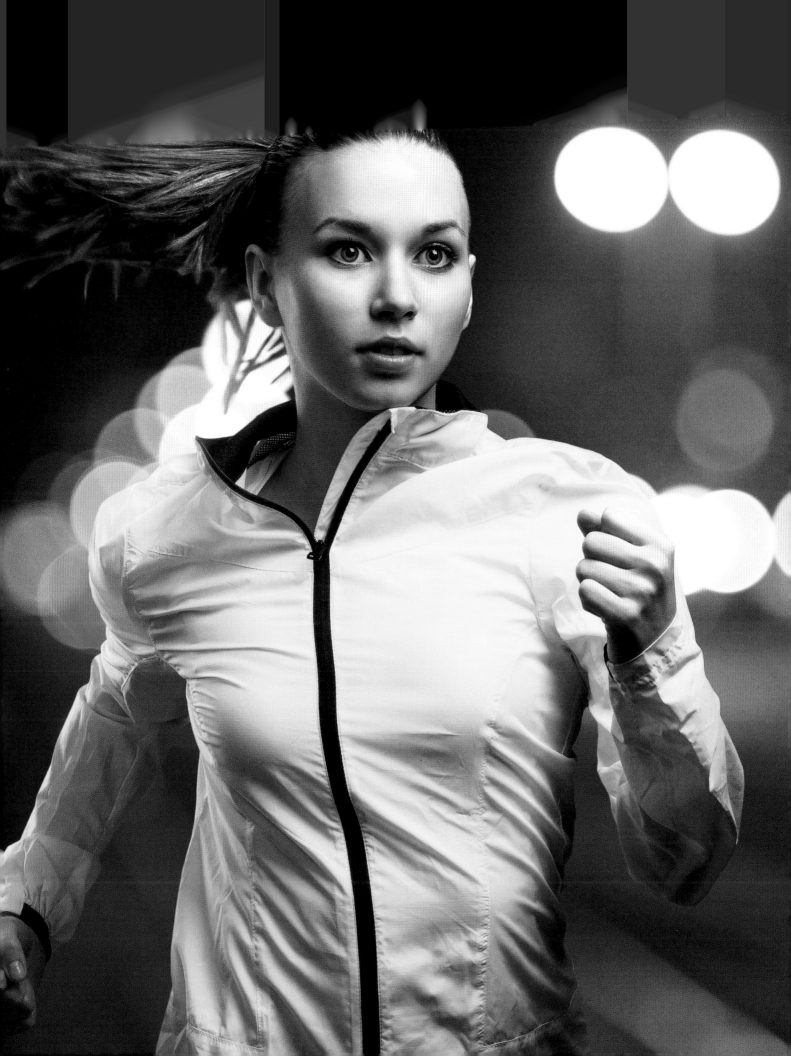

ESSENTIAL KIT

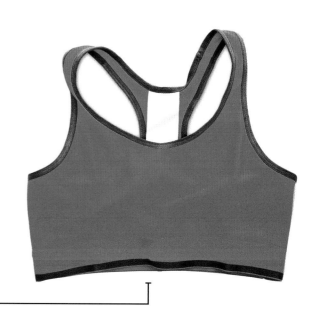

SPORTS BRA

A supportive sports bra is essential for female runners, regardless of how fast or slow you run. Make sure you have a high-impact level sports bra meant for running and not just general exercise. If you don't have a supportive bra, your ligaments can stretch, resulting in premature drooping of the breasts. Change your bra every 40 washes.

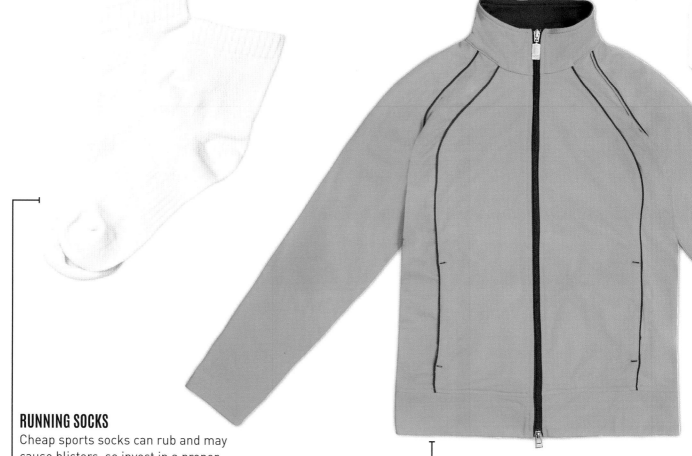

RUNNING SOCKS

Cheap sports socks can rub and may cause blisters, so invest in a proper pair of running socks that are double-lined to help prevent chafing. This can save you from weeks of painful training or blisters that would mean you'd need to rest and miss out on valuable training runs.

WATERPROOF JACKET

Modern waterproof jackets are very lightweight and they're often high-vis and breathable. Plus they usually have enough pockets to hold your phone, keys and energy gels.

BASE LAYER

With a base layer, sweat is wicked away from the skin to help prevent you feeling the chill and to keep you chafe-free in the cold. They have a snug fit, which means you can wear layers over them without feeling too bulky.

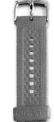

GPS

GPS and running pods accurately measure your current and average running pace, plus the length of your run, which is helpful if you enjoy running a variety of urban routes and need to know the distance you've covered. Although they're not cheap, they are coming down in price. GPS watches lose signal in wooded areas, so inertial running pods can be a better option in these environments. Make sure your device is fully charged up the night before and remember to upload your run to the relevant GPS website to get that all-important breakdown of the stats: distance, average pace and calories burned.

MALE/FEMALE SHORTS AND RUNNING TROUSERS

Shorts will do for most of the year: your legs generate a lot of heat and that means you don't need as many layers on your lower body. But when it gets to the chilliest part of the winter, three-quarter tights or a trackster-type product may save the day.

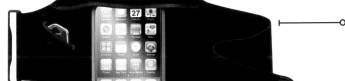

MUSIC PLAYER ARMBAND

Most decent running trousers and jackets have their own music player/phone pocket, but an armband to house your iPod is a useful alternative. It also makes it easy to switch tracks when your ears are assaulted by something that seemed a good idea when you added it to your playlist but really isn't.

KIT EXTRAS

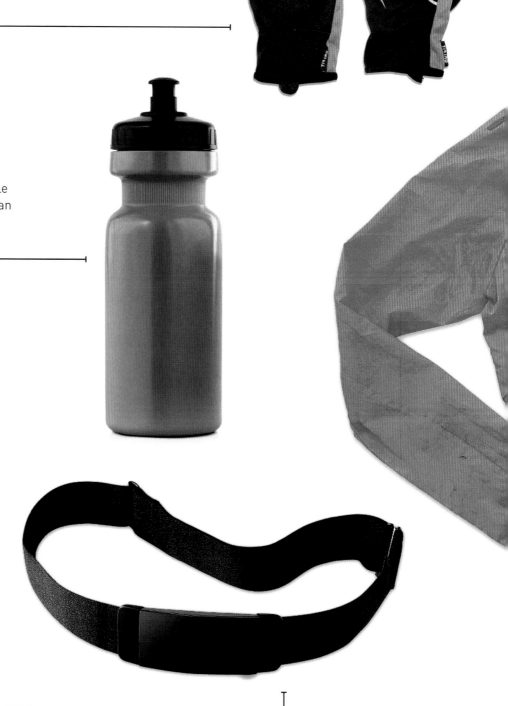

RUNNING GLOVES

You can lose as much as 30 per cent of body heat through your extremities (fingers and toes), so it's important to cover your hands. Gloves should be comfortable, but not too tight.

WATER BOTTLE

Invest in a decent running water bottle that you can grip easily, so that you can drink comfortably without disrupting your running style.

30

HEART RATE MONITOR

Despite popular belief, a heart rate monitor (HRM) is not just a gadget-lover's toy; it's a useful accessory for runners of all abilities. HRMs help take the guesswork out of training, so you know when you're training too hard or not quite enough. They can be very pricey, so make sure you're going to make good use of yours.

RUNNING JACKET

A quality jacket can transfer moisture from your body to the outside world, helping to regulate your body temperature and keep you running mile after mile. Many now also come with handy thumb-holes for comfort and pockets for phones, music players and keys.

RUNNING CAP

Ideal for keeping the sun or rain out of your eyes and to help absorb the sweat from your brow. Look for one that's light and wicks sweat. Other features include a peak with a dark underside that reduces glare.

WAIST BELT

A breathable waist belt is great for storing car keys, energy gels, cash and phone; very handy for those long runs. Try one out if you can as some runners find them uncomfortable.

31

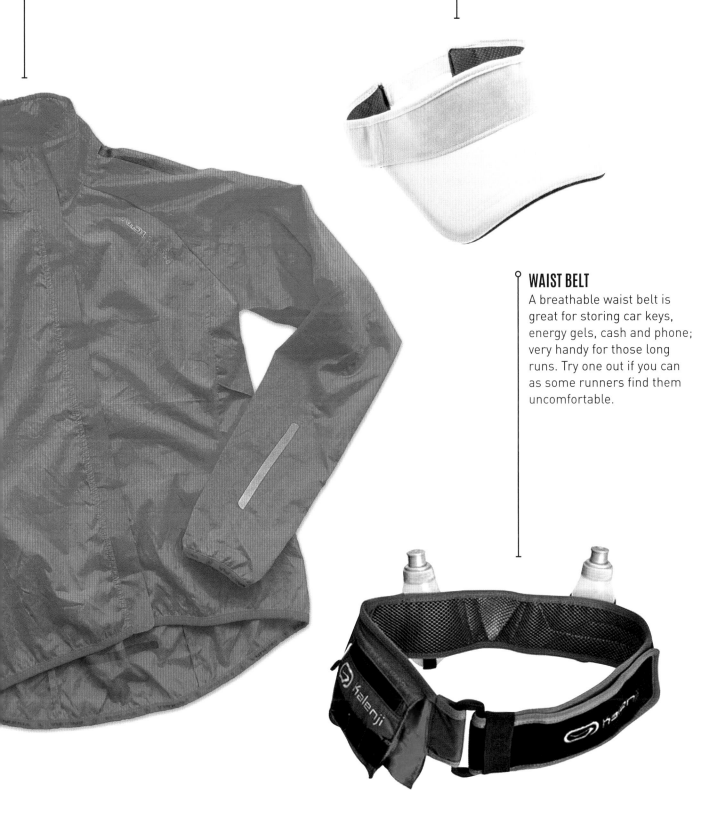

START RUNNING

Don't make excuses to avoid running - you need very little to get started and you can bank miles without breaking the bank.

The beauty of running is that it can be done on – and indeed with – a shoestring. It's important to plan where you intend to spend, as well as shopping around when it comes to races and essential new kit.

GET KIT-SAVVY

American runner and blogger Hollie Sick works in a running shop. "Always ask to see if a running store has older models on clearance," she advises. "Most do and you can cut costs that way. Many local running stores also have discounts for races." Do your research online, too: "Savvy shoppers can find the latest products at the lowest prices on online sites," says Tom Goode, head of marketing at MandMDirect.

Sarah Rowell is the author of *Off-Road Running* (Crowood Press, 2002). She competed for Great Britain in the marathon in the 1984 Olympics, going on to become an acclaimed fell-runner. "Once you know which type of trainer suits you, use websites to buy 'old' models. New models are sometimes just a colour change. I last bought two pairs of my current favourite road shoes at half-price – so tip two is, when you can, bulk buy." Rowell says you need to think about where you need to spend your money. "Shoes, a good sports bra and a waterproof jacket are the top of my list."

Having browsed our kit guide on pp.24-31, be honest. Do you really need all the gear? If you do other sports, you might be able to crossover your kit. Buying T-shirts at the end of summer and winter kit at the end of winter will help ensure you get more for your money. Running and racing off-road have been historically cheaper than road running. Some experts advise investing in two pairs of off-road shoes, which you can rotate. Newcomers may not need to bother investing in a GPS or heart-rate monitor until much further down the line.

DON'T RACE TO RACE

It's so exciting when running comes in to your life and you've done a few races and just want more, more, more! This can quickly end up being very expensive – and may cause a few rows with your partner! If you want value for money, enter a "parkrun", held at the weekend throughout the UK and around the world and completely free. If you want more of a challenge and a great travel experience,

you can enter a fell race for a modest outlay (within the UK). Fell races are not to be feared – anyone can try them and, by the end, you will feel uplifted by the stunning scenery they expose you to. For the price of joining a running club, you can sign up to a season's worth of cross-country races for free. Don't be put off by childhood memories of school runs; the mud is often much more enjoyable as an adult and these races will see your fitness soar.

If you're used to having a personal trainer, it may be tough to give them up but transitioning to a running club can bring a lot of motivation at a fraction of the cost. Most clubs have many different leaders and coaches – all you need to do is click with one. You'll find your running will quickly improve and you'll meet lots of new running buddies, too.

FOOD FOR THOUGHT

You don't need a personal nutritionist. A healthy balanced diet will help your splits (the time you take to run each mile) plummet. Try a free app instead, like MyFitnessPal. At the end of each day you can see what your macros are – that's your carbohydrates, fats and proteins. It also tracks calories and micronutrients and other useful things like sodium intake. There's a good chance that your appetite is going to grow as your running improves. Making your own power snacks is cheap and, remember, healthy, nutritious food doesn't need to cost a bomb. Forget chia seeds and goji berries!

" *The beauty of running is that it can be done on a shoestring.* "

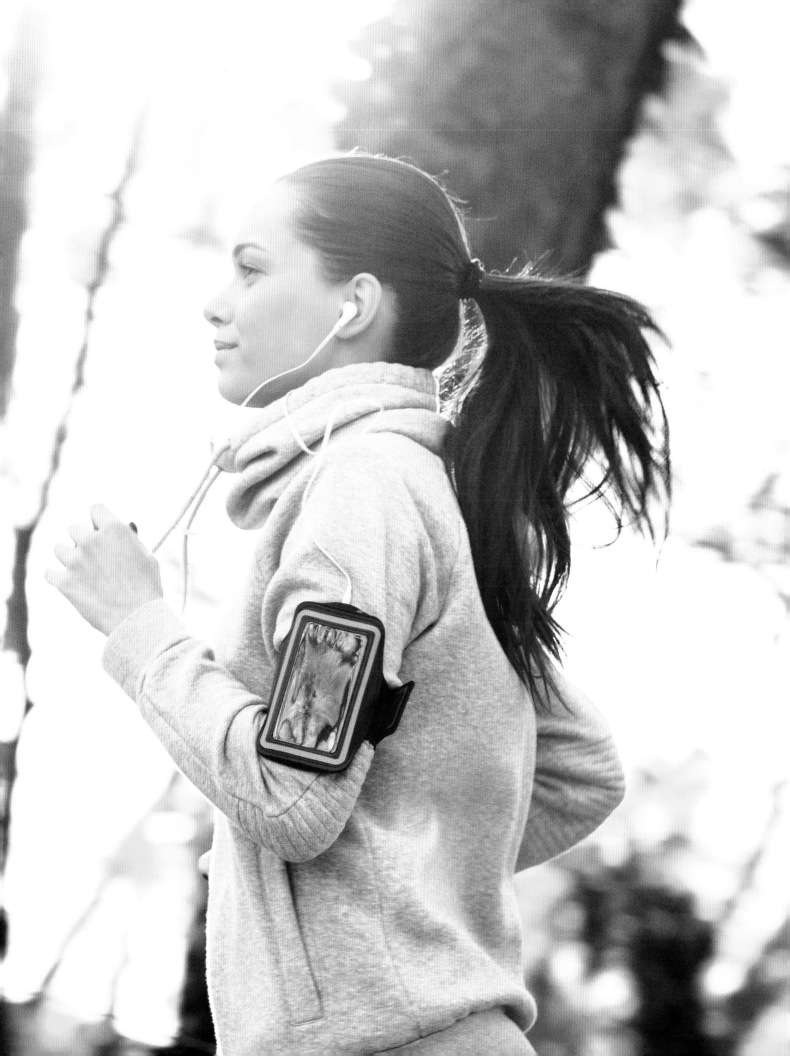

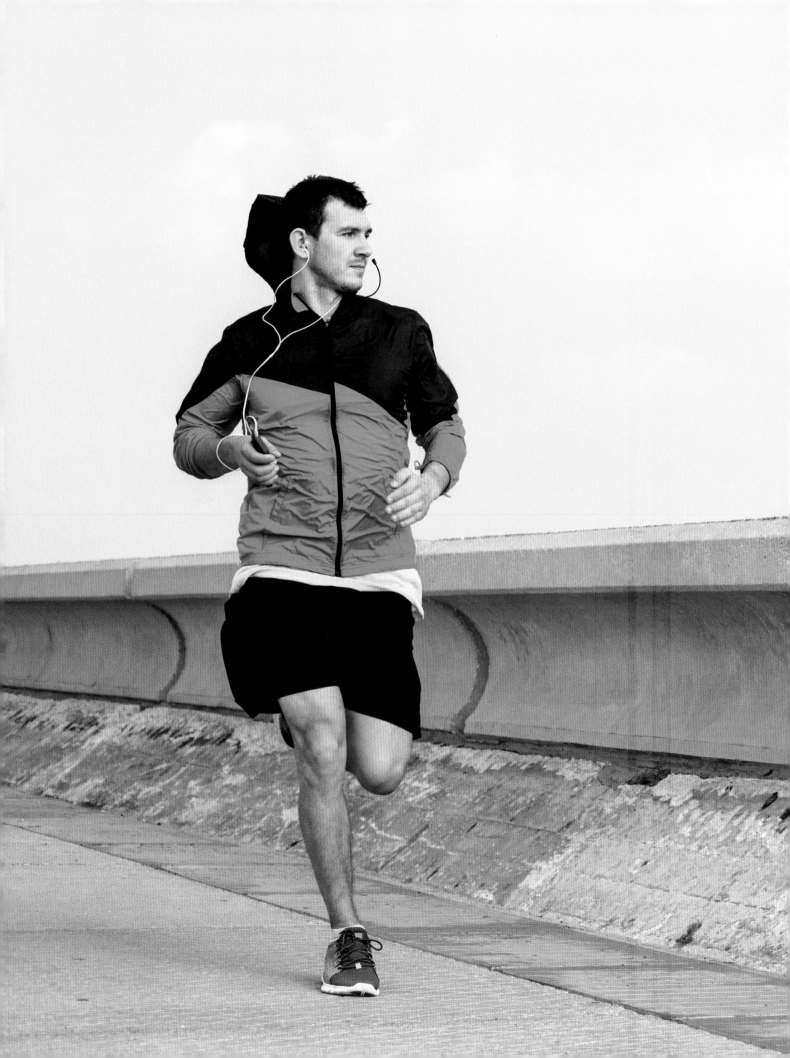

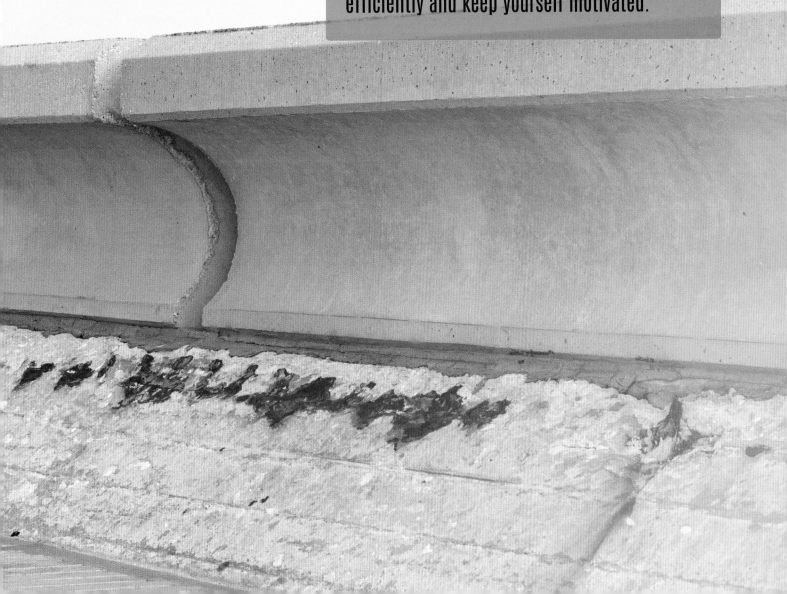

READY TO RUN

Everyone can benefit from looking at his or her running style. Get into good habits from the start, avoid that dispiriting feeling of finding yourself continuously plodding around the same old route with no clear idea of why you're out there, and instead run efficiently and keep yourself motivated.

BEGINNER'S TIPS

Going for your first run is difficult - but it's keeping up that momentum that can be the biggest barrier to fitness.

Habits make the human world go round: we use them for everything from waking up in the morning to going to sleep at night. "We get up at the same time, eat the same food and listen to the same radio station without even realising we're doing it," says Jack Marlow, a sport psychologist. "These learned behaviours become automatic over time. The reason these habits are formed is because they fulfil a purpose in our lives, in the case of morning routines, they prepare us for the day ahead." Clinical hypnotherapist

Peter Mabbutt agrees: "If the behaviour provides some benefit it gets reinforced and repeated. Eventually it moves from being a conscious action to becoming an unconscious, automatic response that we call a habit."

Most running coaches vouch for the fact that running twice a week results in fitness maintenance, running three times a week results in fitness gains and the easiest way to ensure you either maintain or improve your fitness is to turn running into a habit.

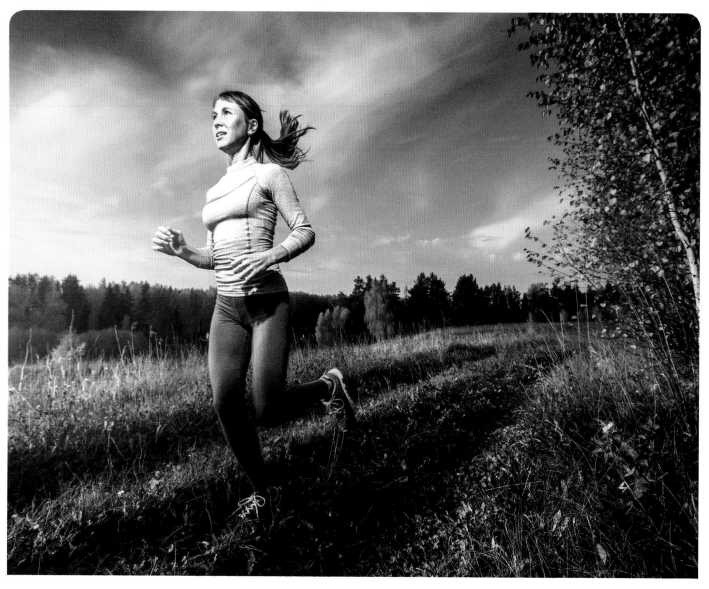

1 LOSE YOUR LIMITING BELIEFS

Transcending limiting beliefs is a very powerful step in achieving what you want, says runner and life coach Jackie Graveney. "You may have a belief that you can't run simply because your sports teacher told you to speed up on a cross-country run. Understanding that this happened many years ago can help you get rid of long-maintained mental obstacles. Creating a new belief – that you can and want to run – will give you permission to move on and act differently, which is the final step to helping you leave that limiting belief behind permanently."

2 SET CLEAR GOALS

"To create a new habit I ask my clients to establish a clear goal of what they want to achieve and why," says lifestyle coach Sally Humphries. "A distinct goal focuses them on where they're going and helps them to determine how to get there. For example, training for weight loss will be very different to preparing for a 5K race or a marathon." NLP (neurolinguistic programming) practitioner Rachel Smith, who's also the joint race director for Saxons, Vikings and Normans Marathons, also says it's important to understand your motivation, as that will make the habit easier to form: "Keep asking yourself, 'And what will that give me?' to drill down to the real nub of what you'll get from running," she says.

Life-coaching's GROW Model is a very useful goal-setting technique that you can use to challenge and focus yourself. Graveney says, "GROW stands for Goals, Reality, Options and Will. Using the four stages, you can establish a 'Goal', such as running three times a week. The 'Reality' of your current situation might be that long working hours mean you can only run once a week at the weekend. Your 'Options' may involve giving up an episode of your favourite soap during the week and getting up earlier on a Tuesday to fit in a run. And finally, 'Will' is all about establishing what needs to be done and committing to doing it in a specified time frame."

3 SEE THE JOURNEY AS WELL AS THE DESTINATION

A common mistake is setting 'dream' goals without considering the process of achieving them, which makes them seem unreachable, says Marlow. "Look at your current long-term goals and then set shorter daily or weekly goals that are realistic and measurable."

4 SEE THE JOURNEY AS WELL AS THE DESTINATION

Hypnosis is a very effective way to create habits. Self-hypnosis will work just as well but requires more self-motivation. "First count yourself down into a trance [deeply relaxed state] by saying the numbers ten to one on ten consecutive exhalations, focusing on relaxing with each number," says Mabbutt. "Then give yourself direct suggestions by listing, step by step, what you will be doing to keep up the running habit. Tell yourself you'll lay out your clothes the night before, what time you'll get up to go, what route you'll follow, and so on. Finally count yourself

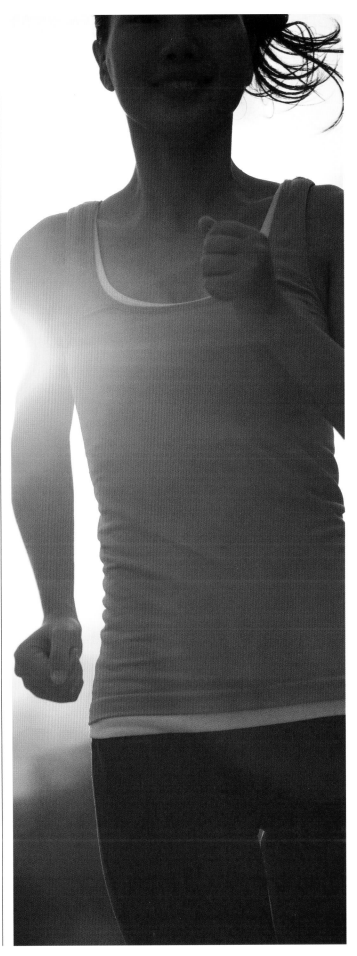

awake by silently saying the numbers one to ten on each inhalation."

You can also try something called 'pseudo-orientation in time' which means creating a three-dimensional psychological reality of the changes you'd like to see in the near future using all of your senses. "While in a trance imagine yourself running regularly, enjoying the feeling of success as you do so, hearing the self-talk that encourages you to enjoy it, basking in the sense of achievement as you develop the new running habit," says Mabbutt.

5 DON'T FAIL TO PREPARE
"Just as your morning routine prepares you for work, a pre-run routine involves behaviours aimed at preparing you for your run," says Marlow. "This can include planning your route, getting changed into your running gear and warming up before every run in a specific order. Doing this before every run will eventually automatically cue your mind and body to get ready to run without having to consciously think about doing it."

6 KEEP YOUR SELF-TALK POSITIVE
List three positive outcomes that running regularly will give you and repeat them to yourself three or four times a day – especially just before you go out for your regular run.

7 CREATE THE RIGHT CUES
"Habits start with a psychological loop that scientists call the 'habit loop'. This consists of three stages. First is the cue (or reminder), that initiates the behaviour, then there's the routine, which is the behaviour itself and then there's the reward, which is the outcome of the behaviour. Usually it is the outcome that drives the habit. Humphries says, "With the reward (outcome) in mind, people use current cues to create a new habit. For example, a daily activity such as brushing your teeth could be used as a cue to getting your kit on to go out for a run in the morning."

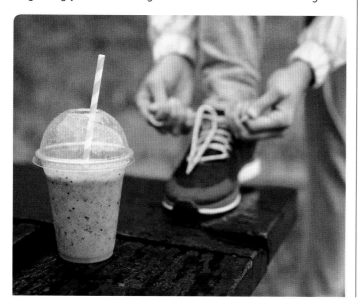

The reward could be the nice long shower you get when you return." Smith says, "With regular repetition of the 'trigger, behaviour, reward' pattern new habits are formed – those automatic conditioned patterns of behaviour that we don't really have to give much thought to but just seem to happen."

PRACTICAL STEPS TO KEEP ON RUNNING

• Find words or photos to remind you of why you want to run and stick them somewhere where you'll see them regularly.

• The more you can plan, the better. Write a plan of the week or weeks ahead: include what days you will run and how long for, what you will do if it rains, what route you will take each day, what and when you'll eat (including shopping for food), what to play on your playlist.

• Set at least one goal for each run. What distance do you want to run? In what time? What do you want to achieve from this run? If your goal is to run every morning for an hour before work, start by running on two or three mornings and build it up. Create a small habit that you can do regularly until it's automatic and then add to it.

• Keep your kit washed and ready for use each day – and lay it out the night before so there's no desperate scramble to find anything.

• Get into performance mode. Change into your running gear as soon as you get home after work or have your gym bag packed by the door in the morning so there are no excuses.

• Find a great runner you aspire to be and model or copy their behaviour – ask yourself, "What would that person be doing right now?"

• Have fun! Running the same route every week can become tedious. Think about how you can make running more stimulating, whether it's through music, spectacular scenery or running with a friend.

• Reward yourself after each run with a cold drink, a smoothie or an invigorating shower gel. This will cause your brain to associate your run with something good, creating a new neurological pathway for your new habit. Every so often reward yourself with something big like new kit or a new pair of trainers.

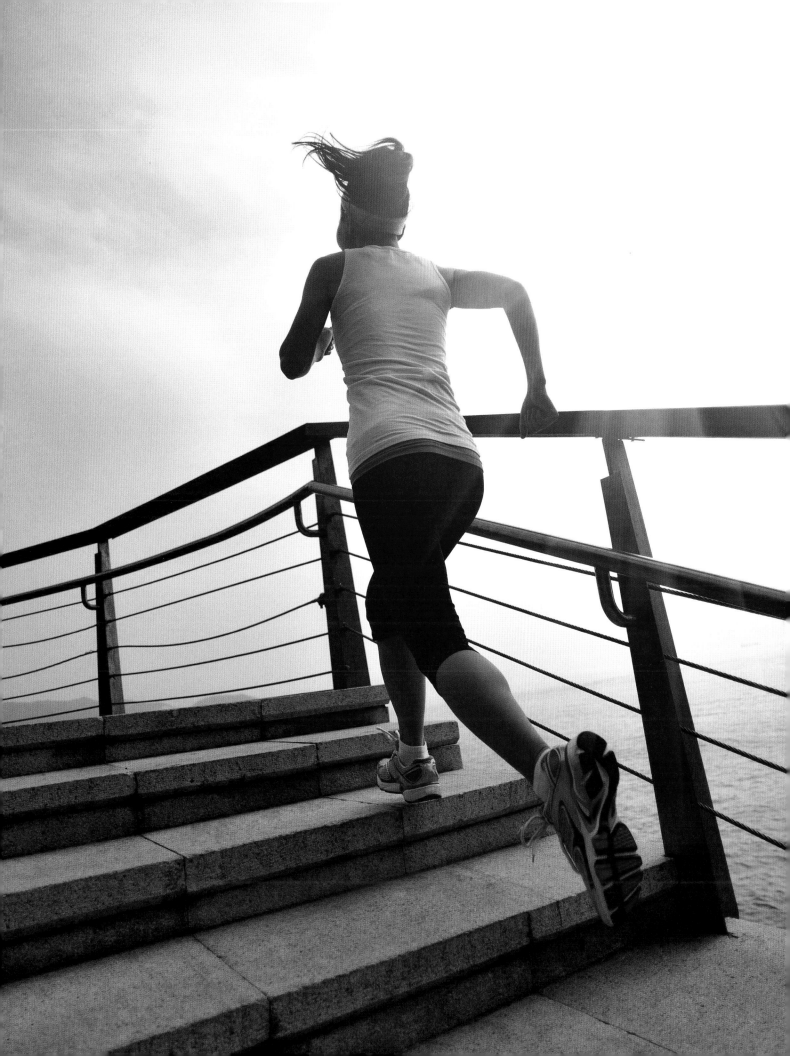

BASIC RUNNING STYLE AND FORM

Good running technique can take you a long way, but first you have to know what that is.

When you get into training for the first time and you start working towards longer race distances, most of your attention will be focused on building up the miles, eating well and getting enough rest, but you should not overlook running technique. Good technique will make you a stronger, more fluid runner and reduce your risk of injury. There are many aspects to technique, including foot strike, arm movement, head position and amount of hip movement. It can be a little difficult to be asked to concentrate on too many elements at once; and the good news is that you don't have to worry about it all at the same time.

The running techniques of elite runners and those at the front of a race vary much less than they do among those runners towards the back of the pack, suggesting that there is significant agreement on the subject of technique for these faster runners. Indeed, if you focus on the mechanical working parts – the hip, knee and foot – of elite runners, you will see body alignment, good, smooth movement and a repetition of that movement over long distances.

FINELY HONED MACHINE
Technique is aimed at both increasing speed and reducing impact. By keeping your hips and ankles in a line with each other and working to ensure your knees do not tend to roll in or wander out, you'll be using all your muscle action

to move forward, rather than putting unnecessary stress on your joints in trying to maintain stability. A running technique for a big distance such as a marathon differs to that employed by a sprinter or track runner. There is less need for a high leg-kick over distance, for example, and it would be very difficult to maintain a high heel-lift for the 26.2 miles of a marathon. Revise, rather than revolutionise, your natural technique, because if you try to change too much at once, your programme may suffer.

RUNNING FORM TIPS

You should be upright – but not militarily erect – in posture, but with your general position moving forwards slightly. It's better to tilt slightly forwards than to lean back.

Relax the muscles of your upper back and neck, which will help keep your airways open for maximum oxygen intake.

Your arms should move back and forth rhythmically, at an angle of 90 degrees. Your arm movement is far more important than you may think, as it will help determine your leg cadence (rate of leg turnover, or the time between steps). Use this influence to your advantage by having relaxed hands. Clenching your fists leads to tension in your arms and shoulders, which saps your energy.

Ensure your pelvis is aligned upright. Try to imagine it as a bowl whose contents you don't want to spill. Sounds weird, but this little tip can seriously improve the fluidity of your running.

Aim to run quietly and lightly, driving forward with each stride, minimising impact and effort but maintaining an even speed.

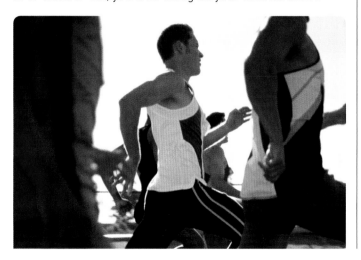

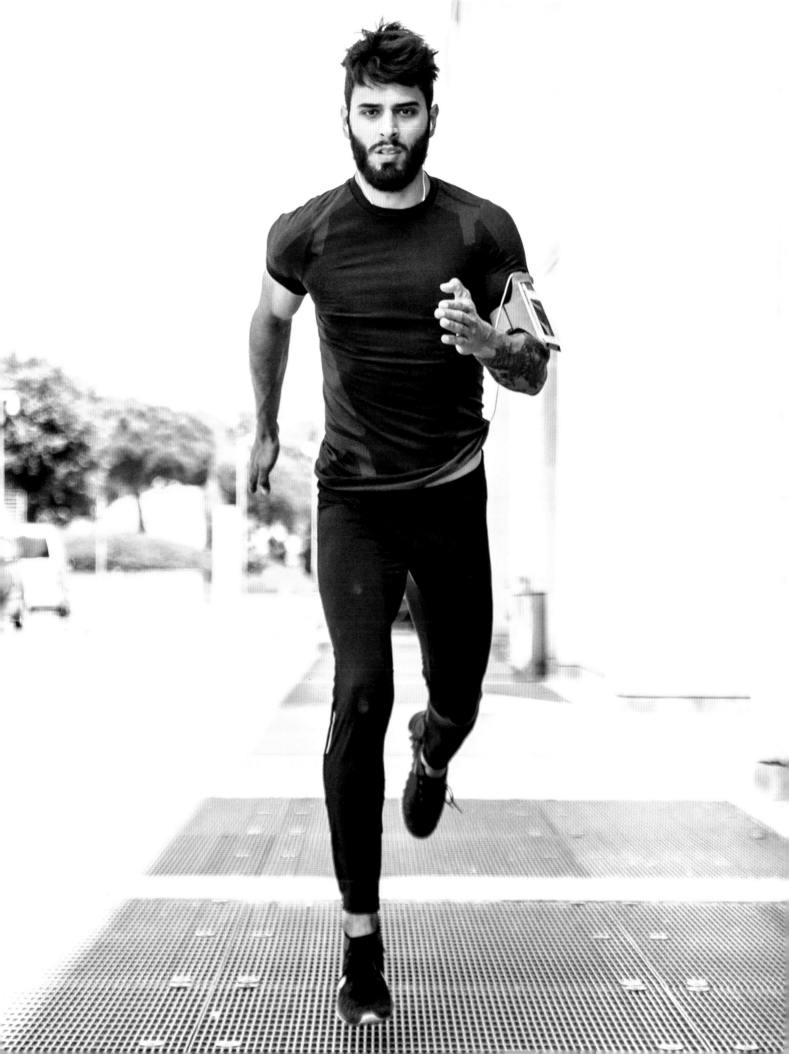

RUNNING DRILL

These exercises will improve your technique:

- **High knees**
  To develop the knee you must drive through each stride.
- **Heel flicks**
  Flicking your heels up to your backside. Concentrate on running tall and fixing your eyes on the horizon.
- **Arm drive**
  Running slowly and in good form, drive the arms forwards and backwards with purpose. Ensure you can feel your shoulder muscles working hard but keep your fingers loose. This not only develops your arm swing, timing and shoulder endurance but also helps you control your posture and pelvis position.
- **Strides**
  Stride out, aiming for longer-than-usual knee drives and more distance between the feet. This develops strength, a good drive off the ground and helps to strengthen those all-important glutes.
- **Hill reps**
  Good for endurance training anyway, but driving hard up a hill develops strength in all the major technique muscles.

Think of these exercises as good warm-up and cool-down tricks to reinforce good technique and improve muscle memory, thereby promoting good form for your next session. Your technique will improve during your training. Developing good technique habits along this journey will bring huge benefits on race day. Remember – good technique is free speed.

IMPROVE YOUR FORM

Better running technique can improve your pace and reduce your chance of injury. Make sure you get the fundamentals right when you first start out.

HEAD AND NECK

DON'T - rock or bob your head backwards and forwards or from side to side, screw your face up or strain your neck.
DO - relax from the eyebrows down. Keep your head level and still, your eyes looking forwards towards an imaginary horizon.
TRY - running relaxed at the end of a run. Spend the final mile consciously relaxing the muscles in your face, head and neck.

SHOULDERS

DON'T – hunch them up when you run, draw them up towards your ears or roll them around.
DO – relax your shoulders and allow them to hang low and loose. Keep them moving freely with the lateral movement of your arms.
TRY – raising and lowering your shoulders, breath out and roll your shoulders gently if you feel tension rising.

ARMS AND HANDS

DON'T – allow your arms to cross in front of your body with each stride or bring them high towards your face. Don't clench your fists or let your hands flap.
DO – remember your arms and legs work together in opposite to keep you balanced and moving forwards. An effective arm action also keeps your legs in check! Try running with your arms moving slowly and your legs quickly – it's very tricky. Swing your arms laterally backwards and forwards by your sides with roughly a 110-120-degree bend at the elbow. Hold your hands relaxed by your sides. Imagine holding eggshells that you don't want to break.
TRY – to allow your arms and hands to drop and roll when you run. Shake them out to ensure they are relaxed before putting them back into lateral motion.

TORSO

DON'T – slouch, twist, lean or dip. Your torso provides stability and strength to your running posture.
DO – run tall. Extend upwards through your spine as you run. Keep upright with your hips, spine, neck and head in a tower-like line. Allow your chest to expand as you breathe. Keep a strong torso with subtle pulling 'in through your belly button' to keep your core muscles stable.
TRY – a regular Pilates class to improve your conditioning and control, especially learn how to master the finer muscle movements.

HIPS

DON'T – let your hips sink or your pelvis drop or tilt. When runners are tired the first sign of poor form is sinking hips. Low hips equal a shortened stride and lower leg lift. Rocking hips should be avoided!

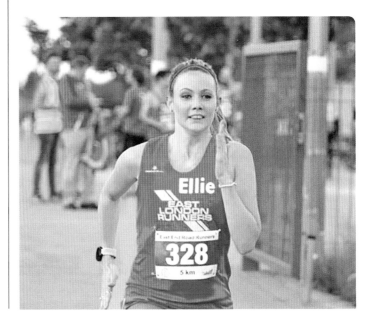

DO – keep your hips high and aligned, facing front. Pelvic stability is really important for good running form. Your hips and torso form the centre of this. Keep your running centre of gravity high to maintain your stride length. Keep your hips stable to give a strong platform to drive from.

TRY – wearing an imaginary baseball cap that sits an inch above your head when you're running. Stretch vertically up elongating your spine and raising your hips to put your head in the high hat!

LEGS

DON'T – let them flail about, flick out wide, cross over, shuffle, or over-stride. Avoid low and high knee-pick-ups or excessive hip flexion.

DO – remember that legs do different things depending on the type of running you're doing. Stride frequency (cadence) and stride length both influence running speed. For shorter, faster running look for a high knee drive, a powerful leg extension, a long reach down with the leading foot and a fast clawing action over the ground with a speedy pull through and return of the opposite leg. For endurance and efficiency, knee-lift isn't as high or as powerful but remains linear with hips driving thighs through under the body and extending with a relatively lower foot carriage under the body.

TRY – short fast sprints. Over 100 metres, accelerate to top speed. As you do, focus on your legs driving through, staying tidy and linear. Get someone to video you to check yourself out!

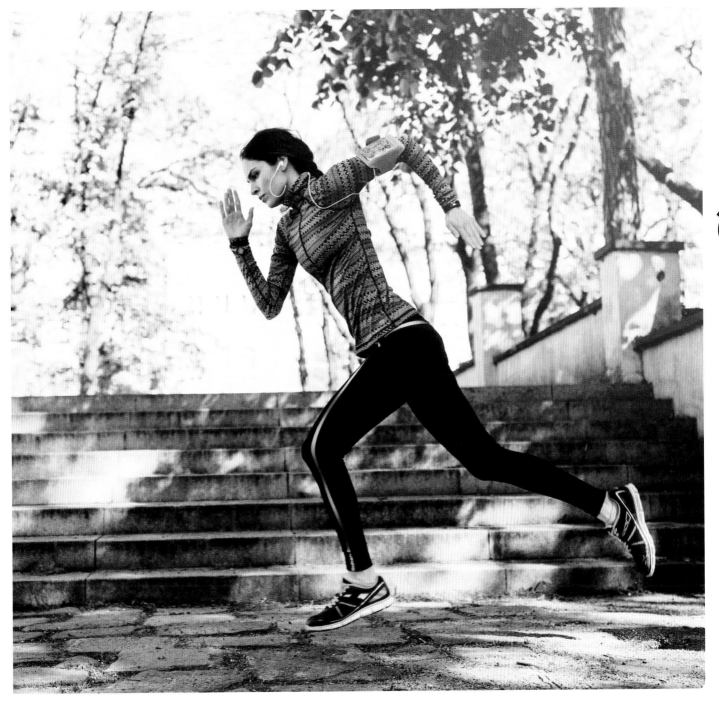

STAY FOCUSED AND MOTIVATED

Mental preparation and attitude is hugely important, as well as knowing how to pace yourself and listening to your body.

When you discovered running, you might have initially found it tough and then got into the swing of it over a period of time. After a while you may plateau and struggle to get faster or simply feel stiff and not be sure why. Equally, if you're training for a long race, it's easy to become daunted. Distance running can be a lonely pursuit and there's also the risk of self-doubt creeping in: that negative voice in your head that pipes up when you're feeling tired, unhelpfully telling you to stop. Developing the right mind-set and using various tactics will help keep you going when you feel tired, or when self-doubt creeps in.

44

WORK ON YOUR MENTAL MUSCLE
Your brain is as important as your legs. Like any muscle, to develop it you're going to have to work on it. Be mindful of what works for you and what doesn't. It's about understanding what you say to yourself and the impact it has on you mentally, as well as restructuring your doubts into something more effective. The best mental strategy for staying motivated during long runs is the one you believe in. Positive mantras can work well for some people, repeating short, positive phrases over to yourself.

When you know you're going to be running for a long time, it's easy to worry at the start about how you might be feeling in a few miles' time. Focus on being in the moment and banish negative self-talk. Acknowledge it when it creeps in, stop it and replace it with your positive mantra.

MIX IT UP
If you're not improving how you want in terms of speed, your training needs to be more demanding. You can't always run at the same pace or cover the same familiar route. Try a different, more scenic route, so that you constantly have interesting things to see, like nature and animals. Your training plan has to be progressive. Increase intensity and incorporate speed endurance work into your plan. That might be interval sessions, or it might be hill running. One threshold run per week and a hill run every one or two weeks will be fine. Do a long steady run once a week. If you've never done intervals, build them into your

running sessions gradually. Start with a few short high-intensity intervals – such as one minute fast, one minute easy – and see how you feel at the end. Threshold runs are a great way to improve fitness. During a threshold run, you'll alternate between shorter blocks of recovery and longer blocks of running at a pace of "controlled discomfort", on a scale of one to ten: you're looking to get to about eight. It's easier to work this out with a GPS watch.

Don't be disheartened if you're not getting much time to train. Try scheduling your runs in advance. Treat them like meetings – mentally commit to them, turn up and do them. Don't overestimate the amount of runs you need to do in a week, even if you're training for longer distances. Three good quality runs a week is fine. One shorter threshold run, one hill run and a longer run at the weekend, where you gradually build mileage, will be sufficient.

"CHUNK" YOUR RUN
Chunking is a tactic that has worked very well for distance runner and Olympic gold-medallist Jo Pavey, who breaks her long runs and marathons into small chunks. "I use mini goals, and focus on my breathing and the rhythm of my legs." Mentally tick each section off in your head, one at a time.

Use your long run to plan your race-day strategy. If you've built up to running more than two hours, planning for a half or full marathon, practice visualising the finish and the completion of your goal. Alternate between "zoning in" – thinking about how your body is feeling and responding to the run – with "zoning out".

> **"** *Alternate between 'zoning in' – thinking about how your body is feeling and responding to the run – with 'zoning out'.* **"**

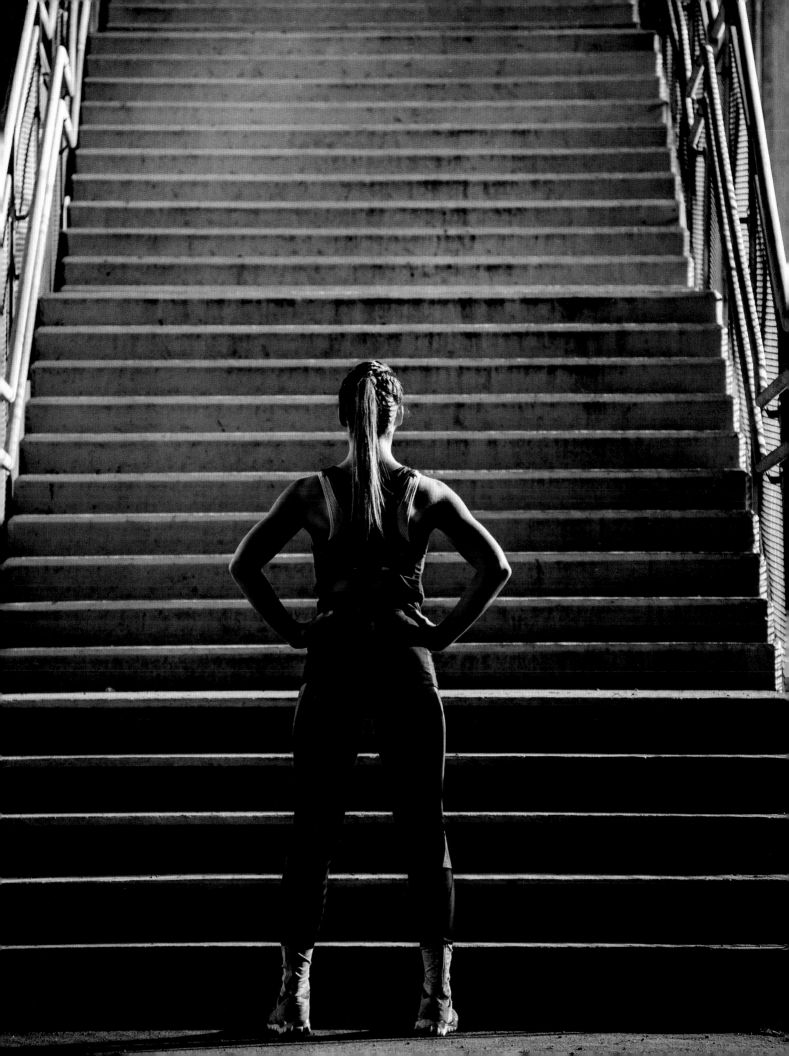

LOW MILEAGE AND INJURIES

If you haven't done enough miles in training for an event or goal, don't try to ignore the fact. Be prepared to walk–run the race. Use mental tactics to get you round. It's about forgetting about your body and thinking more about what's going on outside, which can be easier in event with big crowds all cheering you on.

You may also find that you have a dispiriting number of injuries on a regular basis. Some people are more prone to injury than others. It comes down to the quality of cartilage and also physique and biomechanics. Make sure you've got decent footwear and progress slowly and steadily. The more you run, the more time you need to spend unloading tight muscles, so extra stretching and yoga may help. Sleep is important. It's very easy to cut down on sleep when you're squeezing exercise into a busy lifestyle. But it is during sleep that the body recuperates and reconditions to the rigours of training.

You can look at all aspects of your running if you're feeling stiff or slow – nutrition and hydration as well as rest. Your body may just be telling you something is not right. Speak to a coach who has knowledge of all aspects of training, not just running, and evaluate your current regime. Using a foam roller may help to stretch and roll out the tightness, or see if you can get a massage. Look carefully at all the details of your training, recovery and nutrition so you can experiment with some new strategies – one at a time – to see what might work for you. Look at your recovery time. If your body is aching, it's better to take a day off rather than go out running and cause an injury. It's all too easy to get carried away with a programme. It's far better to do less a week than nothing at all, which is when you will lose your motivation.

CHECK YOUR RUNNING STYLE

"The most common cause of injury in distance runners is poor biomechanics, which is the product of poor strength in some areas, tightness in others and bad technique," says physiotherapist Mark Buckingham. "The trick is identifying these areas. This should be done by a physiotherapist with a detailed knowledge of running technique and the required strength." If you find you are running out of steam in the last half of your distance training or at an event, also check your nutrition. Make sure you're properly hydrated before a race: drink about 500 ml of fluid two hours beforehand and, after the first hour, sip water every 10 to 15 minutes. If you don't think your fuelling strategy holds the answer, take a look at how hard you're running. Slowing down your pace may help over the length of a long run – don't set off too quickly – you may need to look again at your race pace, your threshold running and the amount of hill training that you've built into your schedule.

If you're really struggling near the end of a long race or run, alter your stride length. Reduce your cadence so you're still going at the same speed, but you're taking fewer but longer strides. This seems to help offset fatigue; the theory being you still have some muscle fibres that may not have been used quite as much as the ones that are tired. Finally, you may be underestimating your progress. If you train and get fitter, you will probably still feel the same amount of fatigue at the end but you'll have got there a little bit sooner – you won't feel any less tired.

If you're still finding running difficult, look again at whether you're recovering fully after a session. And check the reverse – are you working hard enough during those threshold runs? If not, you're just putting in loads of "junk" miles, simply going through the motions. Step back and take a look at your training plan and make sure you're not pushing too hard or too little.

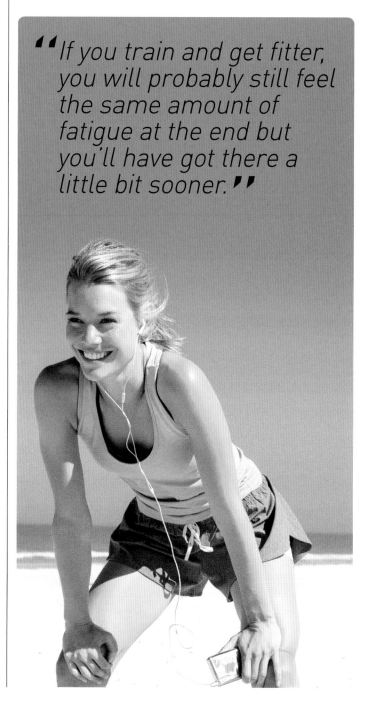

"If you train and get fitter, you will probably still feel the same amount of fatigue at the end but you'll have got there a little bit sooner."

46

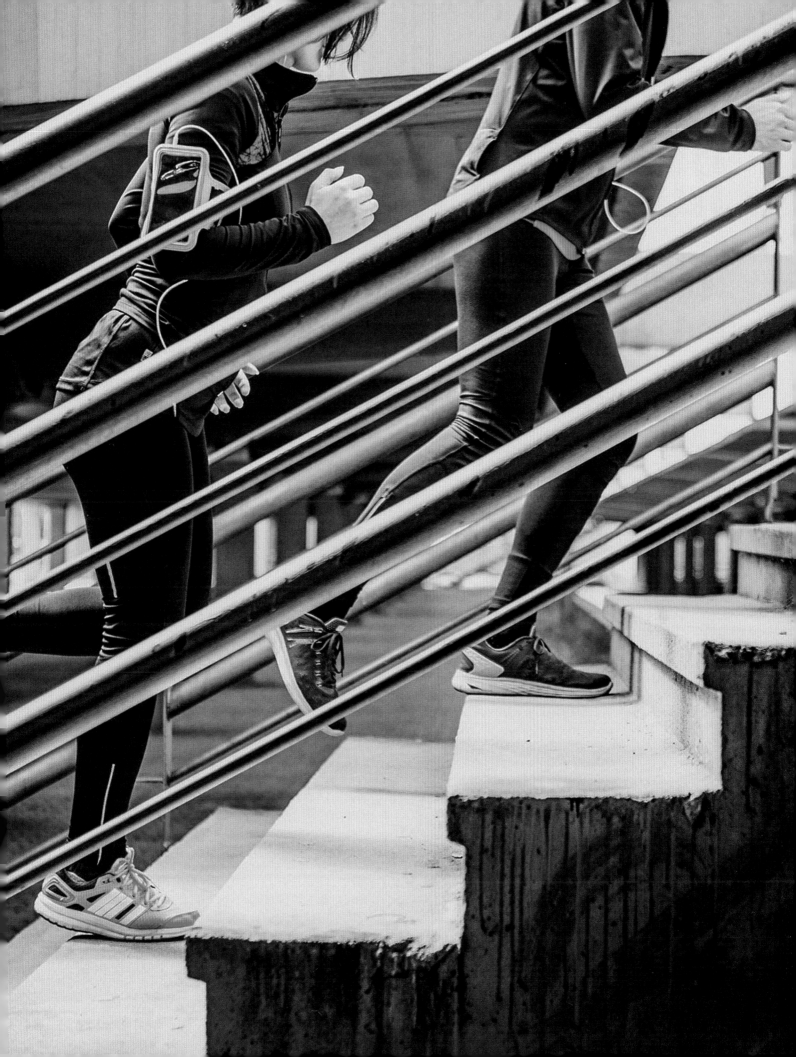

TIPS FOR RUNNING FASTER

Handy hints and a set of four exercises will build your speed endurance as you gain confidence in your running.

48

BIG MARATHON SPEED SESSION

Use this during a key run in your biggest marathon training week, using each of the following exercises, one after another. It looks daunting but hit the right effort levels and it's suitable for anyone. Separate the threshold intervals with 2-minute jogs and allow 3-minute jogs before and after the marathon pace efforts. Add in a good warm-up and cool-down and you've got a great way to make your long run go quicker!

• 30 mins at marathon pace
• 3 minute recovery jog
• 5 x 4 minutes at threshold pace (2-minute jog between intervals)
• 30 mins at marathon pace

KENYAN HILLS

This is a hill session with a difference. Normally you would use the downhill part as a recovery jog, but the key to this session is maintaining the same effort level throughout. First find a runnable hill that will take you a couple of minutes to ascend. After a good warm-up, spend 20 minutes continuously running up and down the hill, making sure you maintain the same effort level throughout (that means you should be going fast downhill). Your effort levels should be just below threshold; similar to the kind of effort you could manage in a one-hour race.

MARGINAL GAINS

Small changes might, on their own, not seem like much. Combined, though, they can make a huge difference to the way that your running develops. Here are some expert tips that should take you to the next level.

ACTIVATE YOUR GLUTES

Include a set of ten squats in your regular warm-up. "These help activate your glute muscles much earlier on in your runs and they take the pressure off your calves," says running coach Nick Antoniades.

JUMP TO IT

Mini-trampolines or rebounders can help with cross-training, as they're low-impact, being ideal when you're recovering from injury. "They work every muscle in the body at one time and help to strengthen the muscles as well as providing a fun cardio workout," says Becky White, a mini-trampoline fitness specialist.

REFLECT AND RECOVER

A time-out period due to injury isn't all bad news and can actually provide you with the space to reflect. "Start substituting negative thoughts such as, 'This is the end of my running', with positive ones, as well as self-talk like, 'I will recover!', and visualising yourself running again," says Dr Rhonda Cohen, a sport and exercise psychologist at the UK's Middlesex University.

IMPROVE YOUR HILL RUNNING

"The key to hills is to try to keep an even effort across the distance that you're covering," says running coach Gary House. "Focus on rhythm, posture and relaxation. Try to pick up your heels slightly with some hamstring activation rather than driving from the quads and hip flexors."

PROGRESSIVE TEMPO RUN - SIX TO TEN MILES

This is a simple but worthwhile session that fits into any training plan. You can personalise the total distance and target pace to fit your own level. You could easily adapt the following to make a ten-mile run starting at an easy pace and then make each mile faster - with the aim of finishing at 10K pace

FOR SIX MILES
- Mile one slow
- Mile two steady
- Mile three marathon pace
- Mile four half-marathon pace
- Miles five and six 10K pace

PARKRUN REPEATS

This is quite straightforward - run 5K, recover for three minutes and then repeat, a total of four times. It might well sound totally crazy - four parkruns in a row? But, just like any speed session, it's all about getting the effort levels right and then anyone is capable. The 5K efforts need to be run just a bit slower than half marathon pace with an easy jog in between. Obviously, you don't have to do them on your local parkrun course, but I like to know I'm running the correct distance and it always gets me in the right frame of mind using a course I'm used to running fast on.

BE YOUR OWN MASSEUSE

You may already have read about foam rollers in the previous chapter but that's not the only tool you can use to help those aching muscles. "Use a tennis ball to ease tight muscles in the buttock or hip area," says sports massage therapist Maria Pali. "Lie on your back or side, place the ball underneath you and then slowly rock back and forwards to massage the area. When you find a tight spot, hold the pressure for up to a minute or until you feel the muscles release."

RELEASE HIP TENSION

"Tight hip flexors [found at the front of your hips] can alter your pelvis position, putting more pressure on the lumbar spine and causing the gluteal [bottom] muscles to lengthen and work at a disadvantage," says physiotherapist and runner Kathleen Walker. "To stretch your hip flexors, get into a half-kneeling position. Place your back foot on a low step or stool. Shift your weight forward on your front leg until you feel a stretch in the front of your hip on the back leg. Hold for 20 seconds and repeat three times on each side."

TAPE IT UP

There's a school of thought that says niggling pains can be managed using kinesiology tape. This is a simple waterproof strapping over your skin, which allows you full mobility and heals at the same time.

EMBRACE HILLS

"Aim to actually run over the crest of hills, rather than stopping once you reach the top," says Charlotte Purdue, elite GB runner and personal trainer. "Most runners stop as they hit the peak, allowing the lactic acid to flood into the legs. Running over the top will help start the recovery."

ENDURANCE STRENGTHENING

To improve your endurance strength, increase your effort during training. "A session I do with my group, which has proven to be successful, is building up steady 4 x 400 metres, with four-minute recoveries in between, before increasing this to 6 x 400 metres with only three-minute recoveries," says endurance running coach Grace Hough.

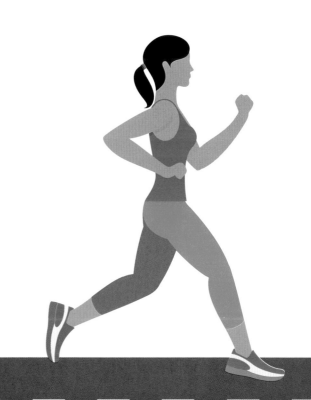

RACE DAY

If you want to have the best possible race experience, it's important to have a failsafe strategy for the weeks, days and hours leading up to your event. Here's how to get it right.

Whether you're about to enter your first race or you've completed a number of events in the past, having a tried and tested race-day strategy and a sound approach to nutrition will stand you in good stead. Planning ahead will give you a much better chance of getting a personal best or simply having a more enjoyable race experience. Being prepared is key to alleviating stress too.

PLAN THE DAY

If you're racing for a personal best then give yourself every possible advantage on the day. Know well in advance what time to get up, what you're going to have for breakfast, what time you'll be eating and all the day's logistics. Know what time you need to leave your home – or hotel if you're racing far away – and what time you need to be at the race in order to avoid pre-race stresses. You can't always control what happens on race day, but you can work out timings in advance to alleviate nerves.

It's natural to be nervous but using the power of the mind will help boost your confidence. Thinking through possible race scenarios and how you would react can help. Write down a few pitfalls and methods of dealing with them. Visualise feeling relaxed, smooth and confident as you cruise around the course.

FOOD FOR THOUGHT

"Two to three days before the race, some runners increase carbohydrates in their diet," says Dr Ieva Alaunyte, a registered nutritionist in sport and exercise nutrition and senior nutrition scientist at Lucozade Sport. "This increases muscle glycogen stores which can be used as energy during a race. It doesn't give you licence to eat anything and everything! Think starchy foods like pasta, rice, potatoes, toast. Close to the race, don't experiment with new foods or products, as it may add stress on the gut. Certain foods may irritate your stomach and gut more than others. Eat a carbohydrate-rich breakfast three to four hours before the race to ensure the food is digested and you don't feel full at the start of your race. Porridge with banana, eggs on toast or breakfast cereal with milk are all excellent choices."

ON THE DAY

Pack up your old kit bag with safety pins, a pre- and post-run snack and a plentiful supply of warm, dry clothes. After the race, your body temperature will drop quickly so it's important to have some dry clothes to change into and something to eat. Don't drink too much water, although it's important to stay hydrated. Monitoring your hydration level using a pee chart is an easy way to achieve optimum hydration. A light straw colour usually indicates you're on the right track. Aim to drink 1.5–2 litres of water on the day. Before the race: start hydrating with a glass or two of water two to four hours beforehand and during the race: drink to thirst, little and often. "For most runners this means drinking little and often, around 4–800 ml per hour," says Alaunyte. "You lose sodium in sweat so replacing electrolytes and energy in the form of carbohydrates may be important for races of an hour or more."

After the race replenish what you've lost. "Drink around two glasses (500 ml) of fluid for every pound of weight you've lost in sweat," says Alaunyte. "A sports drink that provides carbohydrates, salt and fluid can be part of your recovery strategy. A small portion of 15–20 grams of protein (a bar is a good example) is all you need for muscle recovery."

If you're aiming for a personal best, it's hard to know when to put your foot down and when to ease back. Experience is the best way to work this out. That's the fun of racing. The objective of training is to give yourself the right stimulus so you adapt, evolve and get fitter and faster. With racing, it comes down to experience and knowing what sort of shape you're in. With time, you'll work it out.

> *" Being prepared is key to alleviating stress too. "*

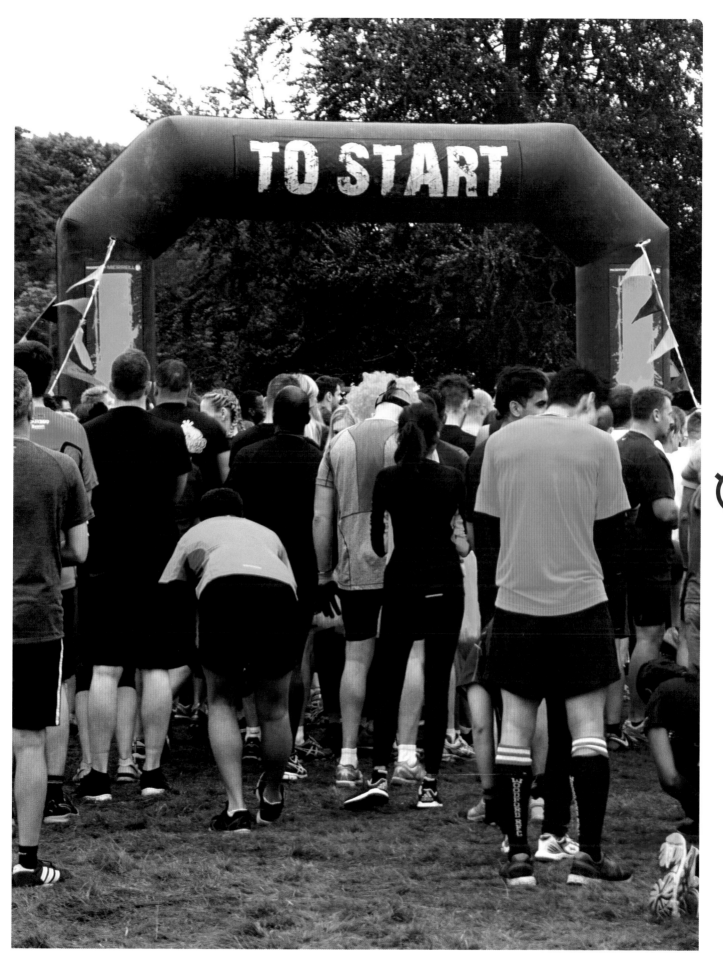

51

RACE PREP

Your first big race day is fast approaching and the fear is rising. If you don't feel ready, don't panic. Everyone has those initial doubts and they're easy to overcome.

Like most people, you probably don't have the time to fit in all the training you want to. You can't change what's past, but what you can do is take an honest assessment of where you are now and what you can achieve between now and race day. Use what you've learned on this occasion to tailor future training programmes.

TRAINING DEFICIT

Examine the distance that you think you're capable of running at the moment and calculate the difference between this and the recommended distance you should be able to complete prior to race day (in a half-marathon, for example, it's 11 miles). Check your diary and see how many weeks it would take you to prepare if you were to continue with the schedule you've been following to date. Either condense your programme to enable you to complete the minimum run in the time you have left or calculate how many miles you'll be able to run by race day and consider how confident you'll feel having got this far prior to the race.

NEED FOR SPEED

Unless you have your heart set on a personal best, don't be too concerned about pace. Just focus on getting plenty of miles under your belt and you may even be pleasantly surprised as to how you perform on the day. If you do need to get round in a specific time, a good strategy is to set aside two training sessions a week for some intensive speed work, in which you gradually increase the time at which you can maintain sprint speed. The more you run at sprint speed, the better able you'll be to maintain a faster average speed. Following a pacer or a fellow runner with a similar pace will also help you achieve your target speed, as you'll be pulled along by the group.

GET OFF THE TREADMILL

If you haven't done enough running outside and spent much of your training on the treadmill in the gym, schedule as much of your training as you can outside. Treadmill running will have given you a good base level of fitness and is useful for accuracy, with different speeds for your interval training, but there is no substitute for outdoor running.

LOW ON LONG RUNS

If you're aiming for a long race event such as a half-marathon, diarise one long run and one medium-distance run each week for the next few weeks. You need to be totally familiar with the feeling of maintaining your running for a few hours and the only way to practise this properly is to get out there and do it. Make sure you have recovery time between long runs and set aside time for plenty of stretching.

UNDER THE WEATHER

If you haven't been running regularly due to bad weather, simply get back into it as soon as possible. You need to get used to contending with whatever conditions you'll face on the day. Test out your kit and your attitude in rain and wind (or blazing sunshine).

CONSIDER DEFERRING

A big part of running a race is what goes on in your mind. If you really think you won't be ready for your forthcoming race, then see if you can defer your entry until the next edition of the event. But, if you feel deep down that, although preparations haven't been ideal up until this point, you're still fit enough to make it round, then push all doubts from your head, get your plan together for the next few weeks and start visualising yourself crossing the finish line and proudly receiving your medal.

"Unless you have your heart set on a personal best, don't be too concerned about the speed you run at."

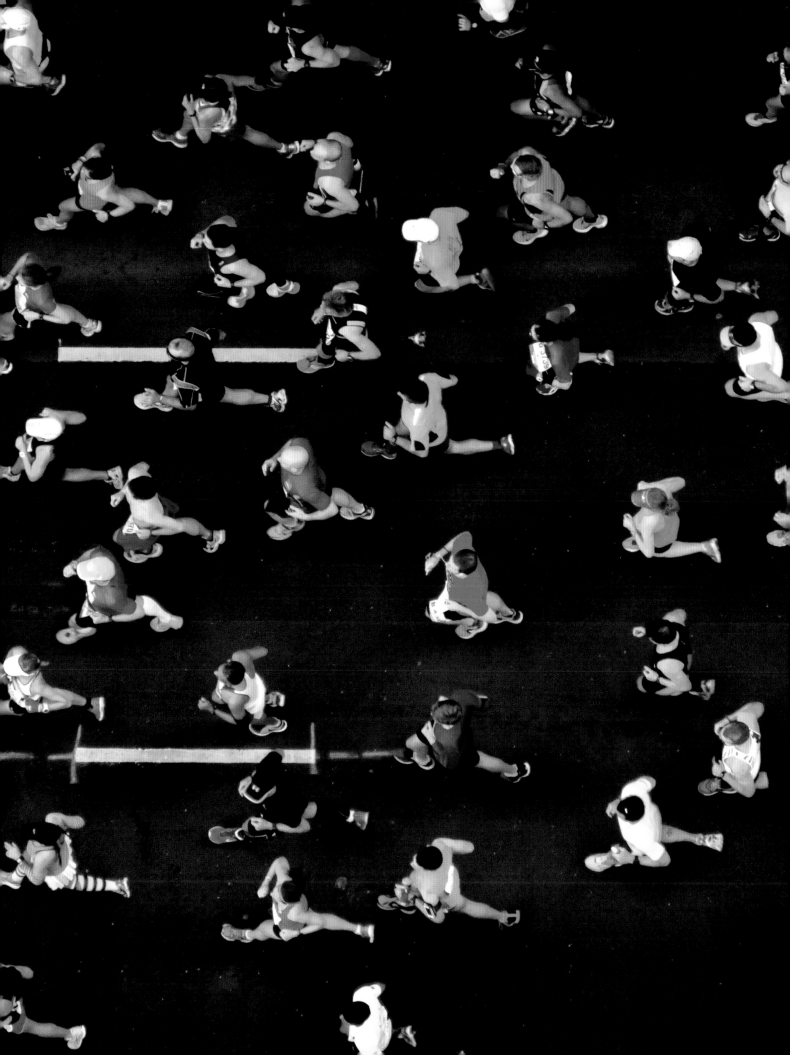

POST-RACE TIPS

Make sure you minimise soreness and recover from your race quickly. The work doesn't finish when you cross the finish line if you want to be sure your body quickly returns to normal quickly.

Running a race, particularly at higher distances such as half-marathons, places several kinds of stress on your body. The muscle tissue broken down over the course of the day will need to rebuild, you need to rehydrate and aching joints need a chance to recover. Here is a step-by-step guide on how to reduce post-race soreness and recover quickly, ready to take on the next challenge.

Straight after the race, don't just stop... walk for about five to ten minutes, as your body doesn't like sudden change and movement keeps your blood pumping around the whole body, preventing it from pooling in your legs. Your body temperature will drop very quickly after a long race, so ensure you get a blanket at the finish, find your bag and get fresh clothes on as quickly as you can (and that's your five- to ten-minute walk organised).

You need to replenish fuel. As we saw in Race Prep (pp.52–53), recovery drinks have all the relevant nutrients in them, which takes away the guess work, so make sure they're in the bag with the fresh clothes. Champagne and beer are not recovery drinks, so leave them alone! However much you want to celebrate, these will cause dehydration and make the pain in the morning so much worse.

EXTRA HELP
You may have access to a gentle massage, which is great, but nothing too deep as your muscles have been through a great deal already. Every hour you need to get on your feet for a few minutes, as your legs will stiffen up and joints need the nourishment gained from movement. This little but regular amount of movement will aid recovery and keep the blood (carrying fresh oxygen and nutrients) flowing to your tired and aching muscles.

Ice baths are renowned for aiding recovery. So, as horrible as it might sound, just ten minutes of sitting in the coldest bath you can cope with will gain significant improvements in your recovery time. Some people even report a pain-free morning after if they indulge in this most sadistic of recovery pursuits. You can also stretch a little and often, just feeling the pull as you hold the position for 30 seconds.

You may not sleep very well after a race. Sometimes your body may find it difficult to switch off, or maybe your aches and pains will wake you up, so it's a good idea to go to bed prepared with water, painkillers, TV remote and a book to take your mind off it all.

THE DAY AFTER
You may feel a bit sore and your leg muscles may be stiff – especially your calf muscles when going down stairs. The amount of soreness you experience depends on your fitness levels and whether or not your body is used to running the distance. Any symptoms should subside after a few days. Doing some gentle exercise, such as walking, cycling in the gym or using a gentle resistance on the cross-trainer, may help reduce stiffness.

You can get back into exercising immediately. Swimming is great – weightless floating with the muscles surrounded by nature's greatest therapeutic tool. This can start after the race itself and continue long into the week after, when your body will still be recovering. The pool is also a great place to stretch muscles, as you will have warmed them up gently and you will leave the pool feeling so much better than when you arrived.

"As horrible as it sounds, ten minutes sitting in an ice bath will gain significant improvements in your recovery time."

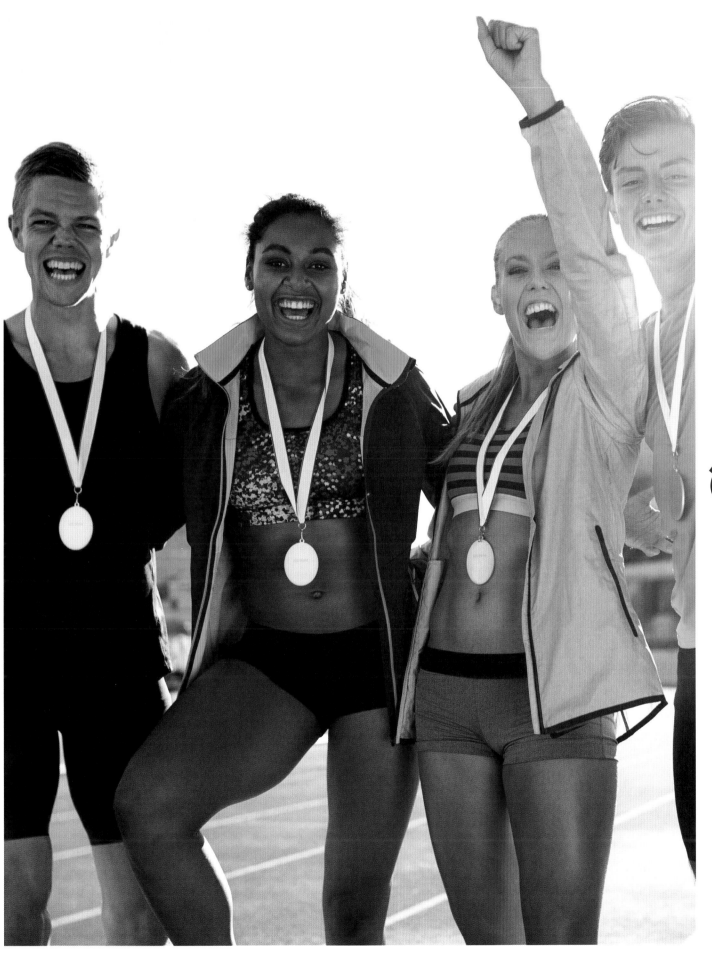

55

VARIED TRAINING

It isn't all about the running. Reduce your injury risk and maintain your fitness with cross-training.

Cross-training is often added to running training programmes to give your body a rest from the high-impact nature of running. It can help reduce the risk of injuries, such as shin splints, while maintaining your fitness and also offering variety and stimulation. Try adding two cross-training sessions a week. The sessions can be anything from attending a class to using the cardio machines in the gym. Try some of the options below to see which suits you best.

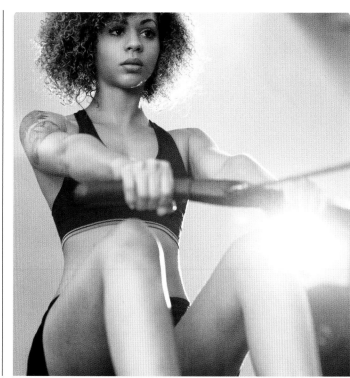

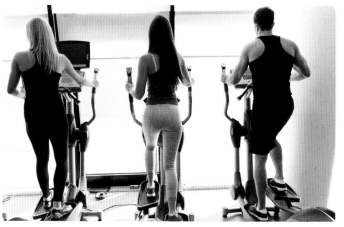

CROSS-TRAINER MACHINE

- **MUSCLES WORKED** – thighs, glutes and upper body. Why is it good for stamina? – The movement you do on a cross-trainer is similar to running but without the impact. It's great if you want to give your hips and knees a break from all the running impact.
- **TRAINING GUIDELINES** – use one of the hill programmes to improve your leg strength. To sprint keep the revolutions per minute (RPM) high to improve your stamina. The RPM settings vary on different machines depending on the size of the flywheel. The faster you go, the more fitness you'll gain.
- **HOW WILL IT BENEFIT YOUR RUNNING?** – The cross-trainer is a great way to improve your cardiovascular fitness without going for a run. The similar movement uses the same muscle groups as running.

ROWING MACHINE

- **MUSCLES WORKED** – upper body, lower body and back.
- **WHY IS IT GOOD FOR STAMINA?** – Although the movement is completely different to running, the rowing machine offers a great cardiovascular workout. By using the smaller muscles in your upper body, your heart rate will be slightly higher than when you run. By training at a higher intensity you will significantly improve your overall stamina levels.
- **TRAINING GUIDELINES** – start by doing five minutes and then gradually increase your workout to 20 to 30 minutes.
- **HOW WILL IT BENEFIT YOUR RUNNING?** Improving your heart/lung capacity will make breathing easier when you run. The less oxygen you use, the longer distance you will be able to complete before becoming tired.

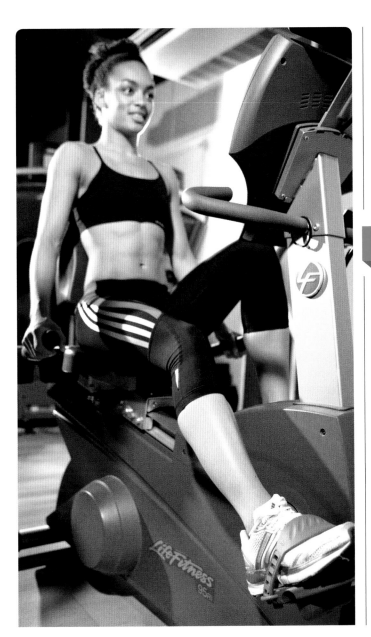

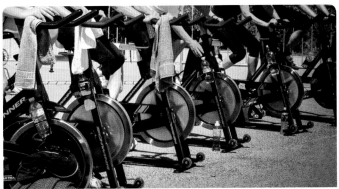

CROSS-TRAINING IN YOUR SCHEDULE

- **MONDAY** – cross-training 40-60 minutes
- **TUESDAY** – run
- **WEDNESDAY** – run hills, sprint or short run
- **THURSDAY** – rest
- **FRIDAY** – cross-training 40-60 minutes
- **SATURDAY** – rest
- **SUNDAY** – long run

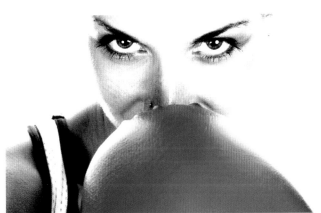

SPINNING/INDOOR CYCLING MACHINE

- **MUSCLES WORKED** – thighs and calf muscles.
- **WHY IS IT GOOD FOR STAMINA?** – Getting the motivation from the instructor, your classmates and the (right) music will help you to push yourself just that little bit harder. The variety in the intensity will also help improve your leg strength and, ultimately, your stamina.
- **TRAINING GUIDELINES** – most spin classes are about 45 minutes, which is the perfect length to fit in a workout if your time is restricted.
- **HOW WILL IT BENEFIT YOUR RUNNING?** – The fitter you are and the stronger your legs become, the easier your run will be.

BOXING OR BODY COMBAT CLASSES

- **MUSCLES WORKED** – upper body, lower body, stomach and side muscles.
- **WHY IS IT GOOD FOR STAMINA?** – By adding a technical aspect to your training, you tend to forget about how you feel and focus more on the task at hand. The instructor will help you get a good workout that will significantly improve your stamina.
- **TRAINING GUIDELINES** – these classes vary a lot, but prepare yourself for a 45-minute class that will not only improve your fitness, but also teach you a new skill.
- **HOW WILL IT BENEFIT YOUR RUNNING?** – The rotational moves in these classes strengthen your stomach muscles, which are important stabilising muscles for running.

HILL TRAINING

You can add something different to your running with a session working on hills. Often neglected, it's a key part of ensuring a broader range in your programme.

If hill-avoidance strategy is something you employ regularly on runs, you're doing your fitness a disservice. Rare is the person who relishes running up hills (it's hard and it can hurt), but learning to embrace rather than avoid hilly terrain will provide you with a natural form of resistance training that will make you stronger.

THE HILLS ARE ALIVE

Scientists have proven hill running to be one of the best ways to tone the lower body and tax the cardiovascular system to its limit. Researchers at the Institute of Sports Sciences in Japan studied the benefits of uphill running and found it activated significantly more muscles in the upper leg and around the hip joint, including the hamstrings (rear thighs) and iliopsoas (inner hip muscle), than running on the flat. All of which is good news if you're looking for more streamlined limbs and a firm bottom.

Other exercise physiologists have shown it to improve the elasticity of muscles and tendons, allowing the legs to run for longer without getting tired. In a Swedish study, twice-weekly hill sessions for three months resulted in a 3 per cent improvement in running economy (how efficiently you use oxygen while running), the equivalent of running at least a minute faster over a five-mile route. "Because it's so taxing, hill-running works the cardiovascular system harder," says Louise Sutton, head of the Carnegie Centre for Sports Performance and Well-Being at Leeds Metropolitan University. "Your heart has to work overtime to meet the increased demands that come with fighting gravity."

DON'T CLIMB EVERY MOUNTAIN

At first, introduce one or two hills to your regular routes before introducing a weekly hill session consisting of eight to 12 repetitions up hills, followed by a jog back down. Vary the incline, distance and terrain as often as possible.

"To be effective for aerobic and strength training, a hill should take at least 30 seconds to run up, but they can take as long as two to three minutes," says marathon coach Bruce Tulloh. Hills toughen you up physically, but are also tremendous for mental training. Every hill you climb makes you feel you've achieved something – and you have.

HILL TECHNIQUE

• As you reach the hill, shorten your stride a little and try to keep to a fast and efficient rhythm. You may find your pace slows, but put in the same effort as you would on flat ground. Try to maintain your tempo by listening to the pace at which your feet hit the ground.
• Don't lean forwards from the waist, as this reduces the involvement of your hamstrings. Keep your head, shoulders and back in a straight line over your feet.
• Use a light push-off with each step and lift your feet a little higher than normal. Imagine lifting your knees as you would when climbing stairs. If a hill gets steeper, keep shortening your stride accordingly.
• Propel yourself with your arms. Keep your elbows bent at a 90-degree angle, pushing directly backwards with each stride (pumping your arms too far forwards simply wastes energy), so that your hands almost brush your hip bones.
• Once you reach the summit, any pain will miraculously disappear. Employ this mental tactic in a race and you could amaze yourself by overtaking dozens of people who stop prematurely, believing the ascent has made them run out of steam.

"For aerobic and strength training, a hill should take at least 30 seconds to run up."

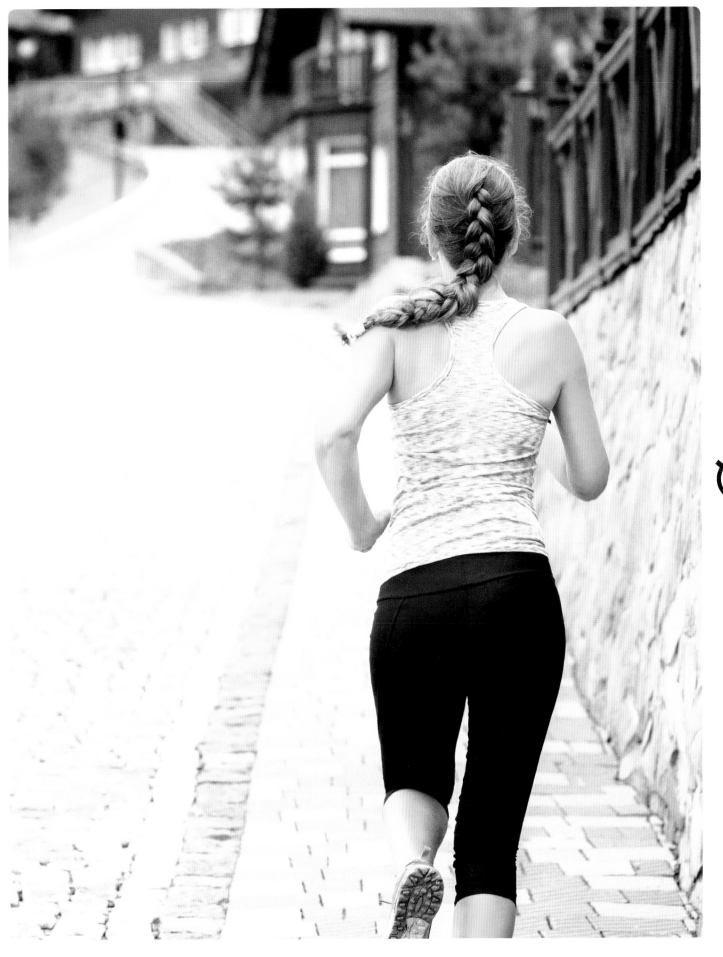

INCREASE YOUR MILES

As you increase your mileage each week, the amount of time you'll need to spend running will naturally increase, too. Beat boredom and make the most of those long runs.

Many half-marathon runners sign up because they love the atmosphere on race day. But alongside the anticipation of the amazing sense of achievement you're going to feel on the day is the risk of being bored out of your mind during long training runs. When you reach the final stages of your training, where long runs can last up to two hours, you could be forgiven for getting fed up at some point, especially if you're pounding the pavements alone.

Adopting a positive mind-set and training your mind to focus on other things will help make those long runs more tolerable. If you feel bored during the early stage of your run, then do what we often do when someone mentions a topic you don't want to talk about – change the subject. Ask yourself questions about the route you've perhaps never thought about before. Try one of those positive mantras. Counting steps is a technique used by Paula Radcliffe that makes you more appreciative of your surroundings.

PARCELS OF MILES
Breaking down your run into separate chunks can also help. If you're going for a ten-mile run, don't think of the remaining nine miles when you complete mile one. Split your run into achievable sections of time or distance. Remember that running is a great way to solve a problem or generate new ideas, so use your mind to distract yourself and resolve issues. If you have a problem, or you need ideas for a new project at work, search for inspiration while you run. The time and space that running offers can improve the quality of thought. Take a few moments to define your problem clearly before you set out, then just let your mind take over while you run.

Running a variety of routes will also help take on different surfaces too. Off-road running is good for building strength and you can keep yourself occupied by concentrating on your orientation and footing on uneven ground.

BUDDY UP
Running can be a solitary pursuit if you choose, but it certainly doesn't have to be. If you want to run with someone, make sure they're a chatterbox. You shouldn't be running long distances at a speed at which you can't enjoy conversation and a partner could make those longer distances fly by. If you're a member of a running club, look for people who love to digress and enjoy telling lots of anecdotes in addition to a main story.

If you're tempted to stop, first question your thinking first. Identify the reason for feeling you can't go on. If it is because you are not performing due to tiredness or illness, then it's important to listen to your body and have a rest. If you want to stop because you are finding it too hard, then you are running too fast and need to ease back. If you want to stop during a session that is intentionally tough with high intensity levels, don't stop, push through it. Think about how rewarded you'll feel at the end and how much stronger you'll become as a result of this type of session.

If you still can't overcome the boredom of long runs then there is also a lot of benefit to be had in splitting the distance. Run in the morning and then go out once again in the evening to achieve your mileage.

60

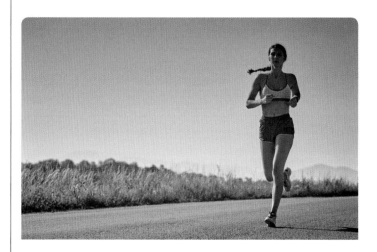

"Counting steps is one technique used by Paula Radcliffe that makes you more appreciative of your surroundings."

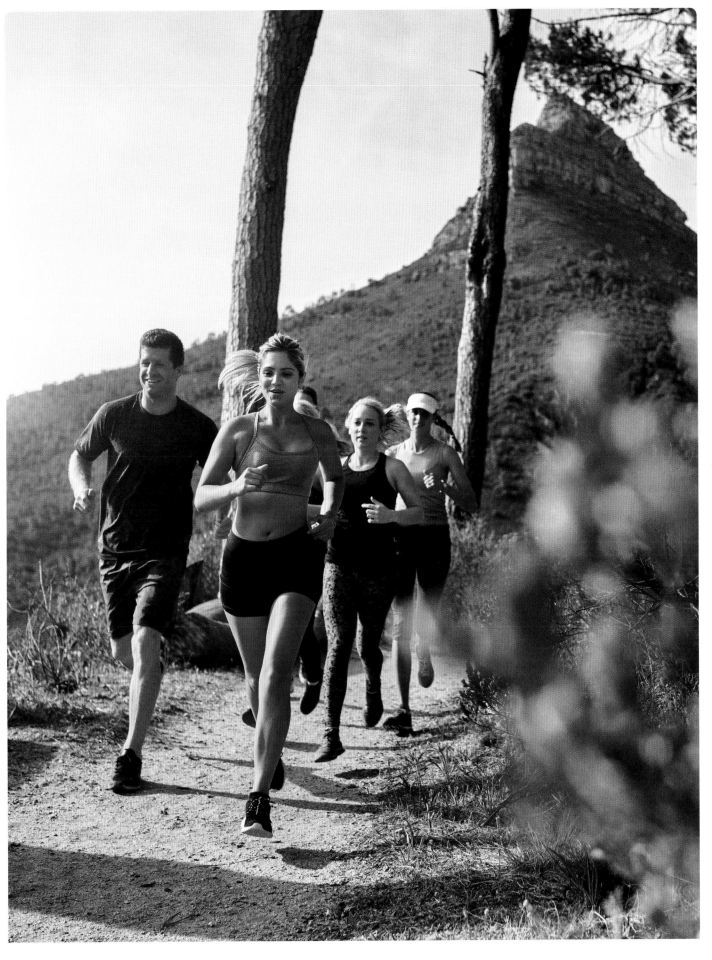

TRAINING MORE EFFICIENTLY

You can pack a surprisingly big punch if you focus your training and work intensively.

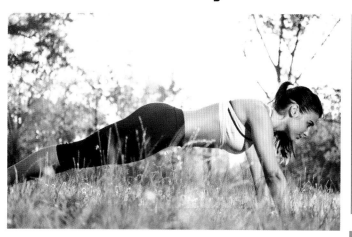

62

Try a lung-busting, muscle-popping, maximum-effort, bodyweight resistance training session that will really test your explosive strength. As you do, make sure that you aren't telling yourself that exercise is something you have to do; start thinking about it as something you want to do. Thinking we have to do something can cause internal resistance, no matter how good we know it will be for us. Exercising our ability to choose makes us feel positive and in control and will mean you're more likely to follow through on your planned workouts.

On some occasions you may want to focus on the other elements of a rounded schedule. Have a great day on the food front, make sure you are well hydrated. If you're working hard make sure you're working effectively by taking regular breaks and concentrate on clearing what's on your to-do list quickly. Then you can relax later and get a good night's sleep. All of this will make your next training session even more effective.

CYCLIST TRICKS
Irish cyclist Martyn Irvine won the points race at the 2013 Track Cycling World Cup with a gutsy approach, proving that the combination of physical preparation, good strategy and quick thinking can be unstoppable. Afterwards he said, "I rode smart for the first half of the race. I didn't want to race too much, but then I started to use my head.

I looked around and other guys were grimacing more than me. I rolled off the front and got in the groove. It was all or nothing." Top man.

Picking a role model is common in the business world. If you're keen for success you'll quickly notice those who hold the positions and have the trappings you aspire to and you'll do what you can to learn from and emulate them.

Looking after ourselves can feel like more of a solo project at times but we can all learn a lot by modelling the success of those who do a great job of combining professional success and good life balance, all underpinned by a proactive approach to wellbeing and resilience.

A SCHEDULE TO FIT IN WITH A PACKED TIMETABLE

- **EASY RUN** - 4 minutes
- **FAST RUN** - maintain pace for 1 minute
- **SQUAT JUMPS** - to failure
- **FAST RUN** - maintain pace for 1 minute
- **LUNGE WALKS** - to failure
- **FAST RUN** - maintain pace for 1 minute
- **PRESS UPS** - to failure
- **FAST RUN** - maintain pace for 1 minute
- **PULL UPS** - to failure
- **FAST RUN** - maintain pace for 1 minute
- **LUNGE JUMPS** - to failure
- **FAST RUN** - maintain pace for 1 minute
- **WIDE LEG SQUATS** - to failure
- **EASY RUN** - 4 minutes

"Focus on the other elements of a rounded schedule. Have a great day on the food front."

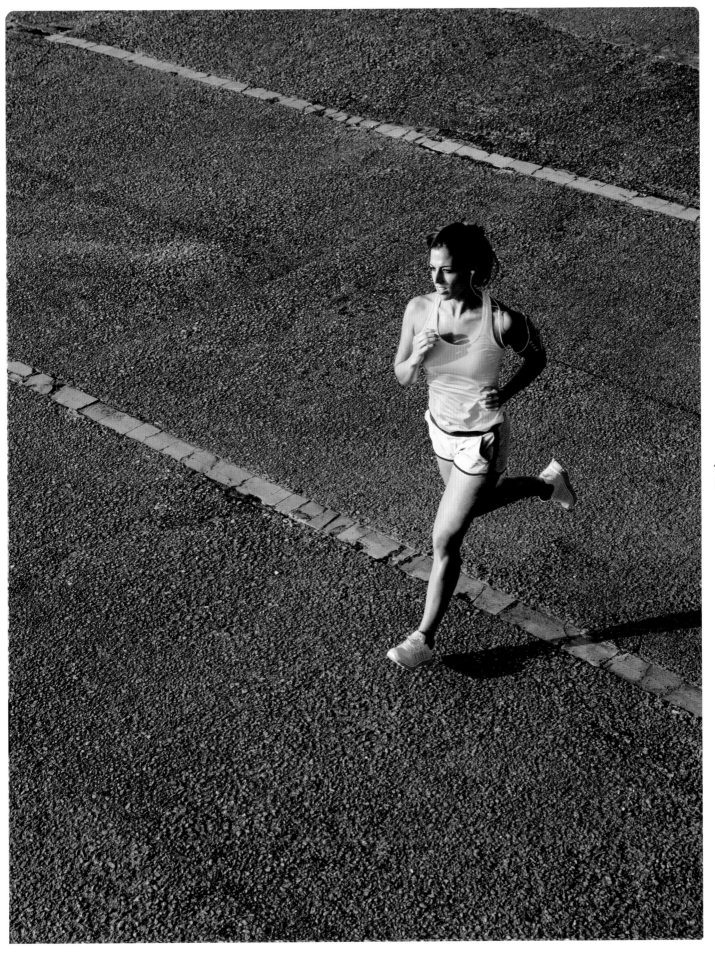

63

ULTIMATE SPEED AND ENDURANCE WORKOUTS

Speed equals distance divided by time. Power equals speed multiplied by strength. In running terms this means that the more strength and power you have, the faster you'll run. For all the exercises here, complete three sets of ten repetitions twice per week in combination with a sprint session.

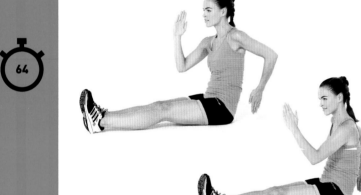

SEATED ARM DRIVES

Muscles used: Arms and shoulders (biceps, triceps, deltoids)

Why do it? Having a good rear arm drive will help to propel you forwards faster.

Technique:
- Sit on the floor with your legs straight.
- Keep a 90-degree bend in your elbows.
- Keep your hands relaxed.
- Swing one arm backwards until your fingers are next to your body.
- The other arm should be up with your fingertips, level with your shoulder.
- Swing your arms as fast as possible forwards and backwards.
- You will bounce on your bottom if you swing your arms fast enough.

Watch points: Keep your back upright and look forward.

RESISTANCE BAND LATERAL SQUATS

Muscles used: Outer and inner thighs, bottom (abductors, adductors, glutes)

Why do it? Strengthening the supporting muscles during the running stride will reduce muscle fatigue.

Technique:
- Tie a resistance band around a pole or secure object to form a loop.
- Stand with your left shoulder facing the pole.
- Place your right ankle inside the resistance band loop.
- Step sideways with your right leg.
- Perform a squat.
- Step back to the centre position.
- Complete one set before changing over.

Watch points: keep the resistance band behind your fixed leg.

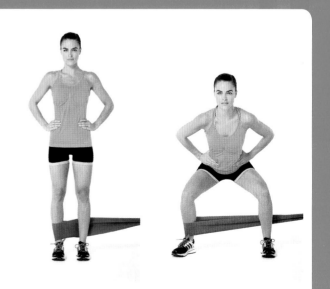

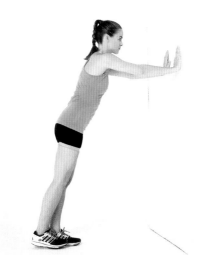

CLAW DRILL

Muscles used: Hip flexors, back thigh (psoas muscles, hamstrings)

Why do it? This exercise exaggerates your running stride, helping to strengthen the muscles.

Technique:

· Place your hands against a wall and keep your body at a 45-degree angle.
· Keep your arm straight.
· Lift one leg up until your thigh is parallel to the ground (high knee).
· Pull your toes up (dorsiflex).
· Explosively push your foot down.
· Swipe your foot backwards and bring your heel up to kick your bottom.
· Bring your leg forward and repeat the move.
· Complete one set on the right before changing over to the other side.

Watch points: To increase the intensity, place a weight on each leg while doing your calf raises.

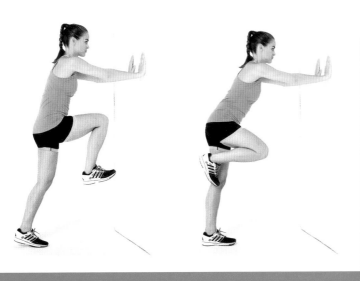

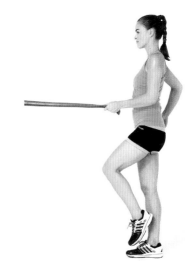

SINGLE-LEG SQUAT WITH SINGLE-ARM ROW

Muscles used: Front thigh, bottom, upper back, core (quadriceps, glutes, rhomboids, lats, transversus abdominus)

Why do it? Performing the running motion with extra resistance will strengthen the muscles and improve your speed.

Technique:

· Tie a resistance band chest-height around a secure object.
· Hold the edge in your left hand, ensuring that there is some tension on the band.
· Balance on your right leg.
· Simultaneously squat with your right leg while pulling the resistance band backwards with your left hand.
· Pull your hand back until it's next to your body in a right angle.
· Return to the starting position.
· Complete one set before switching to the other side.

Watch points: Tighten your core muscle to aid your balance.

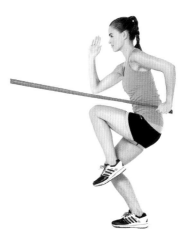

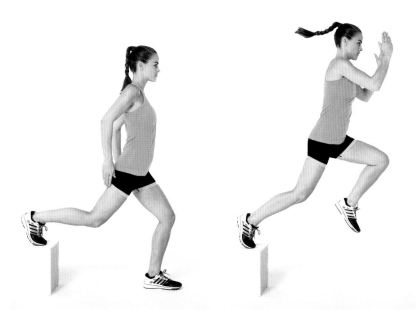

SINGLE-LEG LUNGE JUMPS

Muscles used: Front of thighs, bottom (quadriceps, glutes)

Why do it? This is a great exercise to improve strength and explosive power.

Technique:
· Place your right leg behind you on a step and stand on your left leg.
· Bend your left knee to perform a lunge.
· Explosively jump up.
· Upon landing go straight back into the lunge.
· Complete one set before changing.

Watch points: Tighten your core muscle to aid your balance.

66

WEIGHTED SQUAT JUMPS

Muscles used: Front of thighs, bottom (quadriceps, glutes)

Why do it? The more explosive power you have, the quicker you can accelerate and the faster your speed will be.

Technique:
· Stand with your feet slightly wider than hip width, holding a weight in each hand.
· Bend your knees to perform a squat.
· Explosively jump up.
· Repeat the move as quickly as possible without losing technique.

Watch points: Focus on a point in front of you. Don't look down at your feet.

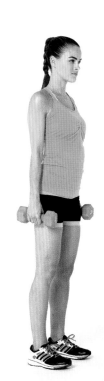
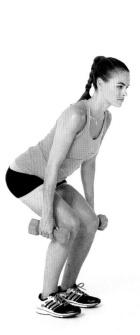
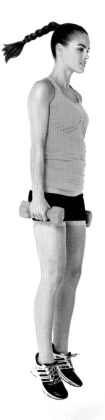

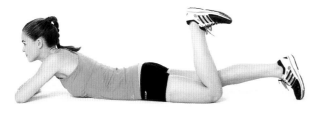

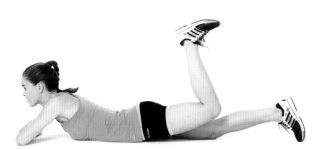

LYING GLUTE LIFT

Muscles used: Bottom, lower back (glutes, para spinals)

Why do it? Activating your bottom during the running stride would help to propel you forward and optimise your running stride.

Technique:
- Bend your left leg to form a right angle in your knee.
- Pull your toes down.
- Lift your knee off the floor without rolling or lifting your hips.
- Complete one set before switching to the other leg.

Watch points: Ensure that you can feel your bottom working and not your hamstring (rear thigh). If you do feel your hamstring, bend your knee more.

67

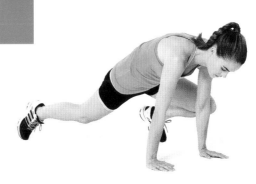

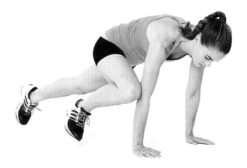

RUNNING MOUNTAIN CLIMBER

Muscles used: Shoulders, arms, hip flexors and core (deltoids, rhomboids, biceps, triceps, psoas muscles, transversus abdominus)**Why do it?** Get your core muscles and legs to work as a unit to improve your speed.

Technique:
- Place your hands about shoulder width apart on the floor.
- Keep your shoulders, hips and feet in line.
- Bring your right knee in towards your right elbow.
- Return to the start and repeat with your left leg.
- Start by walking the move before increasing the move to a run.
- Alternate between right and left.

Watch points: Don't do this move if you are suffering from high blood pressure.

RUNNING FOR BUSY PEOPLE

You may not have much time to devote to running but you can still get race-fit when every second counts.

Nothing beats the inspiration of needing to get fit for a race. Having a date in the diary by which you need to complete a certain distance is a great way to get inspired to run, even when you don't feel like it. Training sessions that might have been ditched in favour of 'a quick drink' after work are more likely to happen with a goal. But sometimes life genuinely can get in the way.

Provided you've got a good base level of cardiovascular fitness and you're not a complete beginner, you can be ready. If you can follow a consistent training plan, you'll be able to reach the start line feeling fresh, fit and confident.

BE CONSISTENT
A lot of runners assume they have to run five or six times a week. This frequency is just not necessary and could lead to injury if your body isn't getting adequate recovery time. Quality is always more important than quantity. Professor Greg Whyte, a sports scientist and former Olympian, recommends lower mileage and good quality training sessions. "What you often find with people is they don't plan their training cycles," he says. "You have got to have a good plan in place and, with that plan, you need targeted, quality sessions."

The training plans at the end of this book (see Chapter 6) have been carefully constructed to build the duration of your runs and boost your fitness without taking over your life. The sessions include one longer run that increases in volume each week and two shorter, more demanding sessions. The shorter sessions will work you harder but are time-efficient.

EVERY ASPECT COUNTS
It's worth spending at least five minutes stretching out the quadriceps, hamstrings, glutes and calves at the end of each run. Hold each stretch for at least 30 seconds. Yoga can be similar, where you're guaranteed to get a good stretch working through poses without rushing.

Running is a high-impact activity, so too much volume can increase injury risk. As we saw in Varied Training (see pp.56–7), a fourth, low-impact cardiovascular (CV) session on the bike, rower or cross-trainer will work your heart and lungs and boost fitness, without the impact. It will also boost motivation. Add some benchmark challenges to your low-impact training to monitor your fitness improvements over time. See how far you can get on the cross-trainer or how quickly you can complete 1,000 metres on the rowing machine.

DON'T PUSH YOUR LIMITS
If you develop a chesty cough or a high temperature, take a rest day. It should be okay to run if you have a light cold – but not if you feel shivery. One or two missed sessions won't affect your fitness. If you do have to miss a few runs, you might feel tempted to try to cram in extra runs during the last few weeks leading up to race day. This can increase injury risk, as you may not be giving your body adequate recovery time. If you're slightly under-trained, accept it and stick to the schedule as best you can.

Above all, run for yourself. Whether this is your first race or you've become a regular runner pushing for a PB, find out what different paces feel like. Discover your own steady pace and your own threshold pace. Don't slow down or speed up for others. It's your race; listen to your own body.

THRESHOLD RUNS

If you want a PB, you want to get used to working at a pace that is not easy but is still controlled. "Doing more miles at threshold pace is key," says running coach George Anderson. "If you can get access to a running track, run hard one lap, then jog or walk for 200 metres then run hard again for another lap."

BUSY RUNNER'S 5K RUNNING PLAN

	MONDAY	TUESDAY	WEDNESDAY	THURSDAY	FRIDAY	SATURDAY	SUNDAY
WEEK 1	Rest	Run 1K	Rest	Run 1.5K	Yoga class	Rest	Run 2K
WEEK 2	Rest	Run 1.5K	Strength training	Run 2K	Rest	Rest	Run 3K
WEEK 3	15 minutes rowing machine; 20 minutes cross-trainer	Rest	Rest	Run 2K & strength training	Run 2K	Rest	Run 3.5K
WEEK 4	Run 2K fast	Strength training	Rest	Run 3K	Yoga class	Rest	Run 4K
WEEK 5	Run 2K fast	20 minutes cross-trainer & strength training	Run 3K	20 minutes rowing machine & strength training	Stretching	Rest	Run 4.5K
WEEK 6	Rest	Run 3K & strength training	Rest	Run 4K	Rest	Rest	Race day: run 5K

BUSY RUNNER'S 10K RUNNING PLAN

	MONDAY	TUESDAY	WEDNESDAY	THURSDAY	FRIDAY	SATURDAY	SUNDAY
WEEK 1	Run 5K	Rest	Run 3K fast	Rest	Strength training	Rest	Run 5K
WEEK 2	Rest	Run 4K fast & strength training	20 minutes rowing machine; 20 minutes bike	Rest	Run 4K	Yoga class	Run 6K
WEEK 3	Stretching	Run 4K fast	Rest	Run 6K	20 minutes rowing machine & strength training	Rest	Run 7K
WEEK 4	Stretching	Run 5K & strength training	Rest	Run 5K fast	Yoga class	Rest	Run 8K
WEEK 5	Stretching	Run 5K & strength training	Rest	Run 7K	Strength training	Rest	Run 9K
WEEK 6	Stretching	Run 6K & strength training	Rest	Run 8K	Yoga class	Rest	Race day: run 10K

TRAIL VS ROAD

Running off-road will not only improve your fitness, but also benefit your mental and emotional health as well.

Which sounds more appealing: jogging in the fresh air of the countryside, with stunning views and nothing but birdsong to disturb the peace, or running on pavements amid the din and traffic fumes? Human beings find the urban environment stressful and the natural world relaxing and reviving. All that concrete, noise and pollution puts us on edge and, over time, it can gnaw at the old grey matter.

Exercise psychologists coined the term "green exercise" to encompass any activity done in nature (including at the seaside, in the countryside and in urban parks). Various studies over the last few years show that green exercise can dramatically improve your wellbeing and reduce problems such as depression.

FIVE A DAY

A study carried out in 2010 by the green research team at the University of Essex, UK, showed that just five minutes of exercise in a green space could significantly boost mental health. A total of 1,250 people took part in the research and participants reported an increased sense of self-esteem and an improvement in mood. Those suffering from mental illness benefited more than most, finding their level of self-worth much improved.

Another study involved a hundred people running on treadmills while looking at pictures of either natural or urban scenes. Only those shown images of a pleasant, rural environment had a large decrease in blood pressure.

In 2006, a study of different types of green exercise found that any form of activity in nature reduced negative emotions (such as anger), decreased tension and improved self-esteem. Experts such as Dr Jo Barton, a researcher in green exercise at Essex, explain the nourishment of green exercise via the "biophilia" hypothesis, which proposes that we have an innate sensitivity to, and need for, other living things – as a result of having coexisted for thousands of generations. "Humans are outdoor animals," says Jo. "Therefore, we feel comfortable, relaxed and connected when we are in nature. There is empirical evidence that spending time in the natural environment is good for you: it improves your mood and your focus. The quality and quantity of contact we have with greenery makes a huge difference to the way we think and feel."

All types of natural environments are beneficial, with urban parks, open countryside and wild woodland all

having a similarly relaxing effect in research studies. However, exercising alongside water was seen to improve wellbeing even more. So, if you can, make sure your running is blue as well as green. Run alongside a river, include a lake, if you can, or maybe even jog on a coastal path.

EMOTIONAL WELL-BEING

UK mental health charity Mind asserts that green exercise should be recognised as a clinically valid treatment for mental health problems. Not only that, but unlike some medication, it has no unpleasant side effects. "Studies show that outdoor exercise can be as effective as antidepressants in treating mild to moderate depression," says Camilla Swain at Mind. "But you don't have to have mental health problems to feel the benefits – all of us can get a mood boost from exercising in a natural environment."

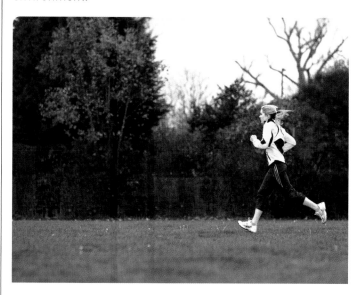

"Spending time in the natural environment is good for you: it improves your mood and your focus."

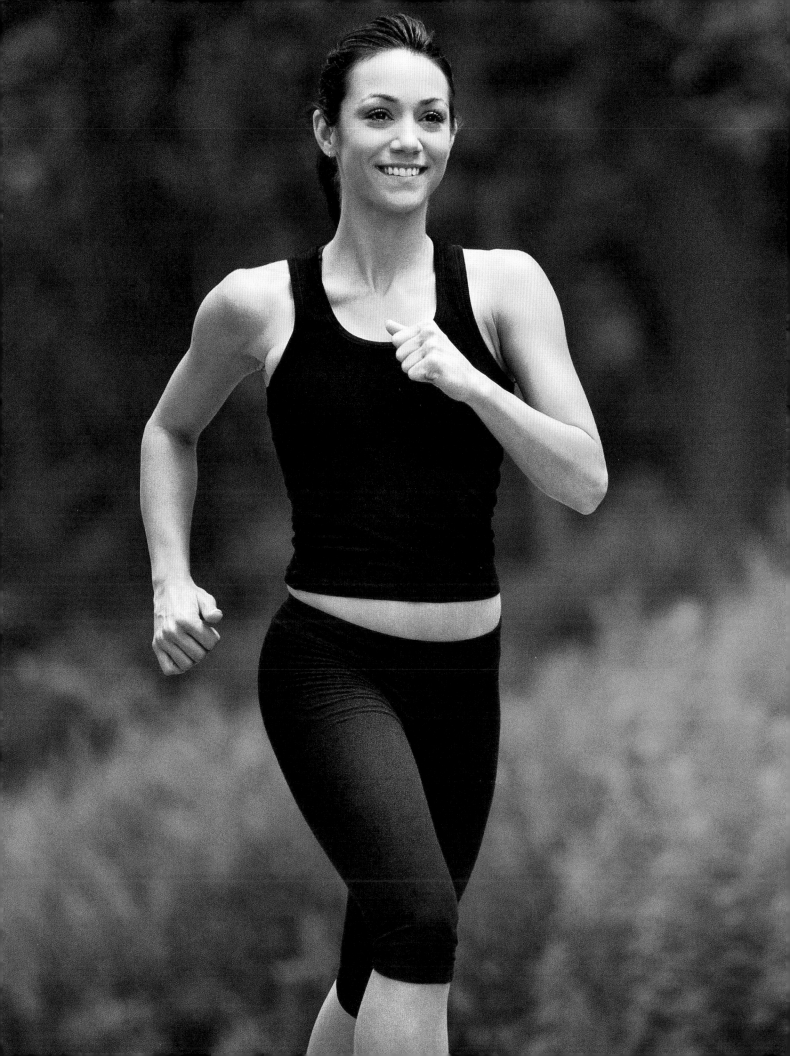

TRACK TRAINING

It can be an intimidating place for the casual runner. But it needn't be: anyone looking to improve his or her speed should turn to the track.

Hitting the track is great for boosting top-end speed, developing your lactate threshold, improving your form and technique, and providing a mix and motivation for your training – and that really does help you run faster.

A track is a fixed distance (400m), meaning it's perfect for understanding pace and effort. It's a very controlled environment, meaning you can structure a specific workout and be able to get feedback on distance and time and see progression as a result of training. Tracks are made for speed, and faster running is good for you. It keeps your motor-neuron pathways sending speedy signals to fast-twitch muscle fibres, keeps your joints, tendons and ligaments more reactive and responsive, and helps with running posture and form.

WHAT TO WEAR

When you first set foot on a track, it can seem like a hard surface. Take your time with any footwear and surface progressions. Just because you're stepping on the track, it doesn't mean you should step out of your normal trainers. A radical move from your normal running trainer to a super light track spike isn't advisable and could result in injury or at least very tight calves.

A lightweight pair of training/racing shoes means that your feet will feel the contact with the track, you'll have better proprioception and you'll be more in tune with your footstrike. Racing trainers are typically much lighter than your robust, heavy, cushioned, supportive mileage shoes so will help you feel light and fast for track workouts. Lighter shoes have also been shown to be more efficient and energy saving. They are, however, less supportive and have reduced cushioning, stability and control.

Running spikes take the lightness and minimalist nature even further. A classic track spike is wafer thin and light providing only minimal protection but increased traction and responsiveness through the addition of a spike plate at the forefoot.

TRACK TECHNIQUE

You don't need to run differently or change your running style when running on the track. However, it is a great place to perfect your posture and form and become a 'tidy'

runner with balance, poise and control.

• Keep your hips high. Run tall. Imagine you are reaching upwards to place your head in an imaginary baseball cap just above you.

• Run confidently. Keep your eyes on a virtual horizon level, head high (not chin up), arms swinging laterally by your sides, increase your leg cadence and your stride rate and look and feel great.

• Relax – don't strain. You don't need to screw your face up in a sinewy smile to run fast. Instead, keep your head, neck and shoulders still, relaxed and in control. Relax from the eyebrows down.

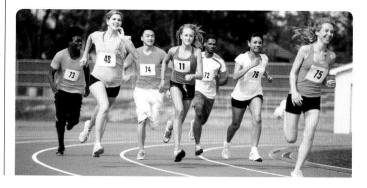

TRACK TRAINING

• RUN THE SHORTEST DISTANCE
On a track this means that you run on the inside of Lane 1.

• KEEP AN EVEN PACE
While running on a road, the course often dictates your pace as you have to navigate left and right turns, uphills, downhills and even wind. However, running on a track is all about learning how to hold a steady pace each lap.

• COMMIT TO IT
Track running takes courage and commitment. Your mind must be ready to invest the effort to in order to reap the rewards. Don't just hop on the track and run around for a few laps. Aim to hit it with purpose.

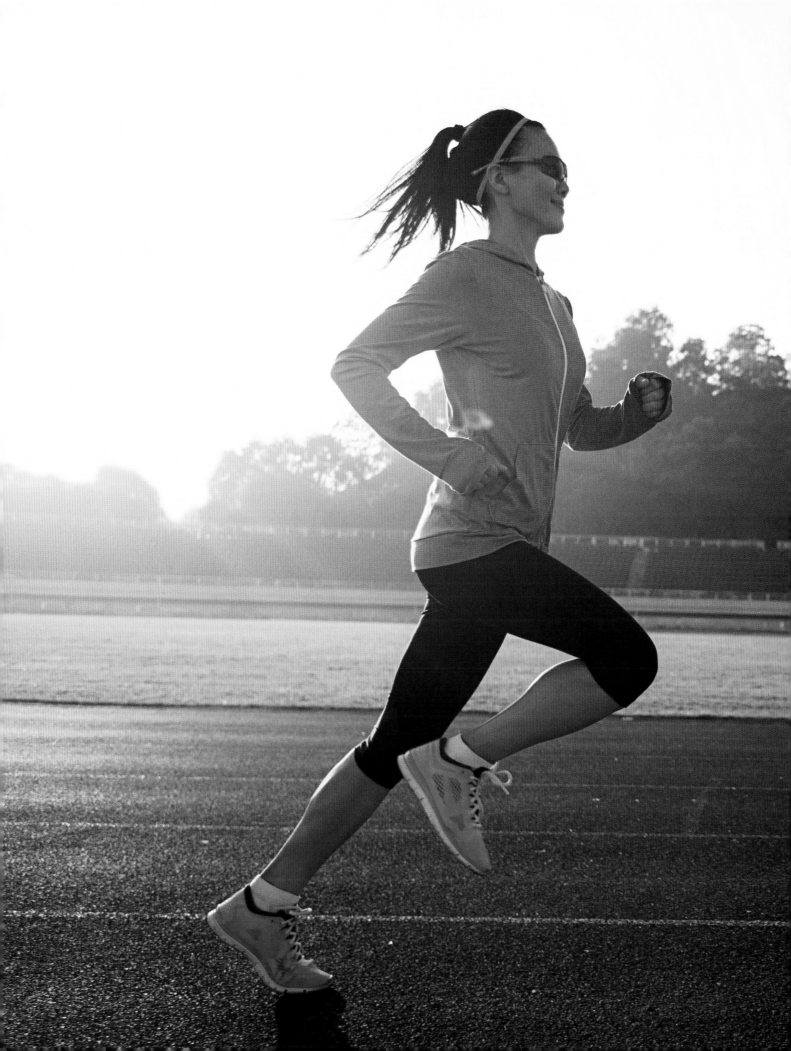

PUSHING YOUR BOUNDARIES

Turning up your mileage should only ever be good for your running, in theory, but that's not always the case.

From the first step of our running journey, we think that further is probably better and our first measure of improvement is how far and how often we're able to run. As a rule of thumb, running three times per week, for 30 minutes at a time, is considered a good level for fitness. But what about when you're managing that comfortably? What happens when your idea of "better running" starts to be measured not just in terms of non-stop jogs or 10,000 steps per day and starts to be about improving your speed or racing longer distances? At this point the temptation is to do more of the same, to keep adding runs to your week until you're hopping out of bed and straight into your trainers on a daily basis without even thinking.

MORE IS BETTER

Running more is a good idea if you want to improve your race performance – up to a point. Running three times per week, especially if you're not fitting in any other training, will only get you so far. So your first step to getting better at any distance is to build up to running five or even six days per week. That not only gives you a better foundation in terms of your aerobic fitness but also allows you to vary your sessions from day to day so that you're training every aspect of your fitness.

Variety is essential to making your higher volume training work. If you are just running the same 30-minute route, at the same "fairly hard" intensity five or six times per week, you'll quickly find that your fitness starts to plateau. It's easy to become demoralised: your pace starts to drop and you just don't want to go out and run any more. You may start running harder or running further on every run – both are shortcuts to injury.

When you're comfortably running five or six times per week, make sure you think about the function of each of your runs. Even if you're not training for a particular event, it's worth mixing up your runs so that your fitness doesn't stagnate.

REST IS BEST

Your body needs at least one day of total rest to recover. People who don't rest are likely to suffer from over-use injuries, such as shin splints or runner's knee. You will begin to notice you're not as energetic as you used to be. You might feel fatigued all day long, but struggle to sleep. You'll constantly feel as though you're coming down with something. Your mood will suffer. Collectively, these symptoms are known as overtraining syndrome – common in elite athletes and among everyday runners like us, who don't have a coach to tell us when to stop.

Your training week doesn't have to consist of seven days. If you're really keen to run more and improve your times, then you could follow the example of elite runners and use an eight to ten-day training cycle, with one day off. Be very careful if you plan to try this though, and only do it if you're still consistently seeing improvements in fitness with a weekly cycle.

TWICE AS NICE

Training twice a day may sound excessive, but most of the very best runners in the world use this tactic. One daily run will always be at a low intensity level, with the other devoted to building speed, strength or working on running technique. Start with an easy run one day; double up the next day with one short, easy run and one speed-work session; go easy the next day; then double up the day after that with another short light run and some hill reps. This is not for inexperienced runners. You need to have built up to it over the course of a couple of years. There are plenty of easier ways to improve before we need to start double-dosing: strength and core training, regular physio checks and targeted speedwork are all likely to be more beneficial.

> *"Training weeks don't have to be seven days. Elite runners use an eight to ten-day cycle."*

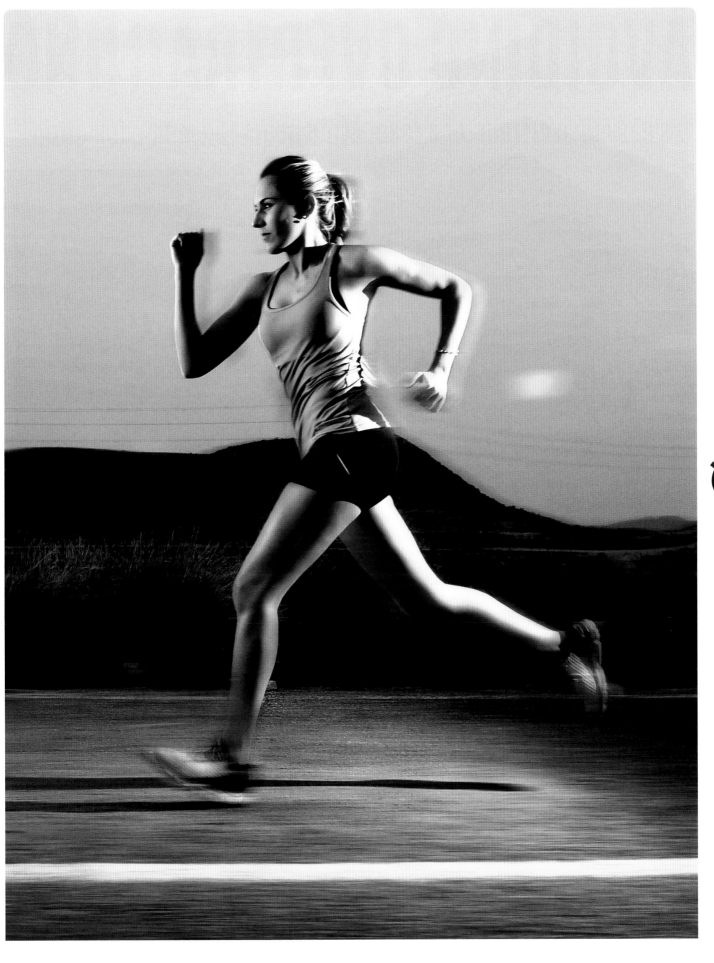

AVOIDING OVERTRAINING

It's easy to overtrain for a race. Avoid doing too much, too often.

Remember that training sessions are for challenging your body and pushing the boundaries of your capabilities, but it's the period following those training sessions when your body grows fitter and stronger, as it adapts to the workload. Overtraining can rob you of the opportunity for this adaptive progress to take place.

The easiest way to avoid overtraining is to follow a structured training plan – devised by yourself or an expert – and to keep a diary of training notes so that you can regularly monitor the results of that plan. Some people argue that the symptoms of overtraining emerge following too many long runs or taking on regular tough sessions back-to-back, with little recovery time, but this pattern of training need not necessarily have negative consequences.

Indeed, training at a high volume or intensity can be a great way to improve your ability in a relatively short space of time. The most important thing is to keep sight of the fact that your recovery time should be directly related to your training workload. If you are planning to push yourself hard in training, make sure you plan at least two recovery days per week and more if your regular progress review suggests that your body needs additional recovery time following a challenging training period.

BE PATIENT

Be realistic about the time it will take you to prepare for a marathon. Even if your training plan is designed to just get you to the finish line, with no specific time, your objective isn't really to just get round, but to do so without suffering injuries along the way and then needing two weeks to recover.

When selecting your training plan, be honest about your running ability, allow yourself plenty of time to increase your mileage and do the necessary cross training, strength training and flexibility work that will keep you on the road. Then add a few weeks as a contingency for unforeseen work and/or family commitments that may get in the way of your training, or for time off required by any minor illnesses or niggles along the way.

Provided you make this time, you'll be able to offset some heavier training weeks with some lighter periods and the variety in your weekly workload will ensure that you are able to take big steps forward with your running progress and still have time to recover properly.

Every session in your plan should have a structure and a specific purpose. If you take this approach, you won't waste time on unnecessary extra training sessions or running for the sake of it and logging junk miles (owing to a lack of planning, you end up heading out yet again without a goal). If you don't know why you're out there – hill session, interval session, a tempo run or easy jog – you may be wasting an opportunity to rest.

It's often said that running a long race is easy and that the real challenge is training for one. So take your time, plan your approach and focus on the quality of your training. If you do that, the quantity will follow.

76

> *"If you are planning to push yourself hard in training, make sure you plan at least two recovery days per week."*

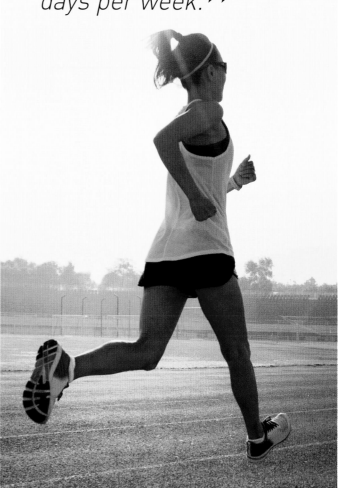

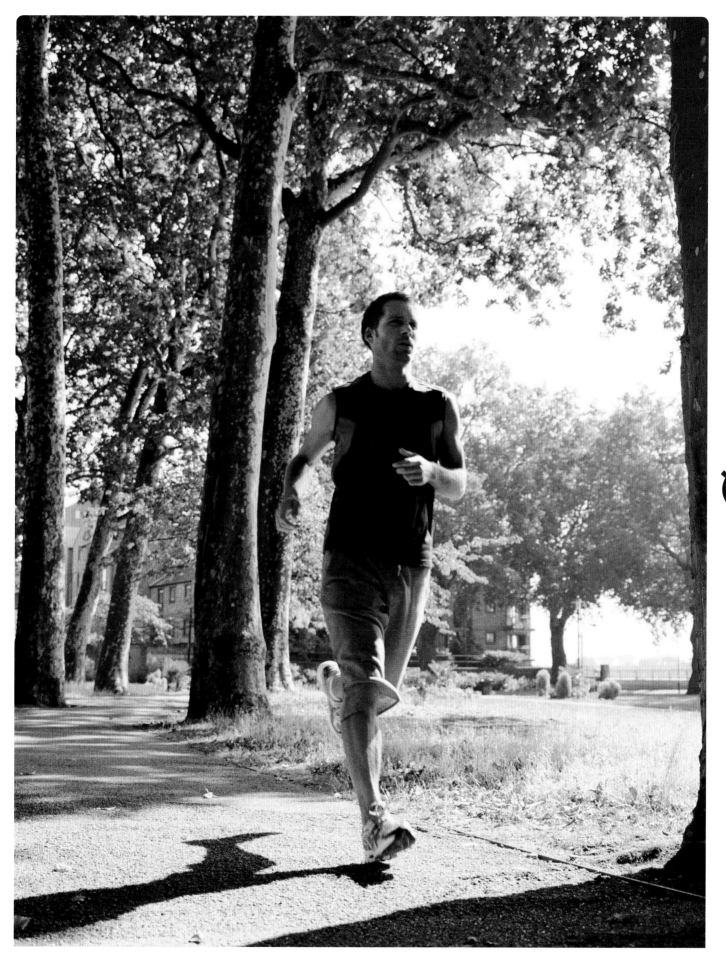

HALF-MARATHON TIPS

Hints to take you from novice to expert as you increase your training distance all the way to the final week before your race.

As you get closer to your race, your mileage will likely be increasing, with your long run increasing in length and perhaps an extra session in your weekly run programme. This can mean missing runs or dragging yourself around your routes if you don't satisfy your body's heightened demand for nutrients to provide energy for training and recovery.

As your body gets used to regular running you can also find yourself struggling to control a ravenous appetite, trying desperately not to eat more calories than you've burned. The long run in particular requires special nutritional thought, as this will have subjected your muscles to a great deal of micro-damage, emptied your body's fuel reserves and placed you in a vulnerable position in terms of your immunity.

KEEP FUELLED

You don't need an energy drink prior to each run, but do ensure your run is timed two to three hours after your last meal. This will leave your body well-fuelled and avoid that uncomfortable feeling you can get if you run too close to eating. If you're planning to run early in the morning you will be better off with 3–500 ml of an energy drink before you head off, but otherwise simply timing your meals and snacks so that you're running at the optimum time will support better performance.

Sip on water throughout the day. Research in the Scandinavian Journal of Medicine and Science in Sports indicates that most of us start running already dehydrated. Increase the amount of water you drink daily, ensuring you are at least taking on eight glasses of water throughout the day. This will also have the benefit of helping with tissue repair after a long run and the added side effect of plumping up the skin to make you look younger, too.

THE 90-MINUTE RULE

Runs over 90 minutes require extra fuel. You should ideally be taking on 60 grams of carbohydrate per hour, mixed into a drink or in a gel form. For example, a two-hour run should be supported with two bottles or one bottle with carbohydrate to be refilled at the halfway point with water and one to two gels to supply carbohydrate for the second half of the run. You'll be amazed how much better you'll feel.

Runners tend to be confused about how much to drink on the run, with research indicating that dehydration

impairs performance and over-drinking can be unsafe. The best way to work out your individual hydration need is to weigh yourself before and after a one-hour run. For every kilogram lost you should be replacing a litre of fluid, so if your weight has dropped by 0.5 kilogram then your hourly need is 500 ml. Simple. Now aim to stick to this intake for every hour of running.

ENTERING THE LAST WEEK

The final week leading up to the race can feel like a period of limbo, where the training is complete but the race isn't here yet. So what's the best way to spend the final seven days before you get to the start line?

It's a dilemma: on the one hand you'll want to sneak in a few extra miles just to top up your fitness level and make sure you won't have forgotten how to run come race day. On the other hand, you'll want to rest as much as possible and this might even include thinking twice about any extra trips to the supermarket.

At this point, there isn't really much more improvement you can make to your fitness level, so your focus should be on resting your body and getting your mind into the right space for race day. That said, it's often a good idea to do one or two short runs in this last week, both as a way of running at a gentle pace just to keep things moving while planning your race tactics on the go. It is also a good way to warm up before you spend a concerted period of time stretching to ensure you're as loose and relaxed as you can be.

RACE-DAY STRATEGY

On the face of it, completing a half marathon simply requires you to keep running for 13.1 miles. While this is true to a certain extent, your task can be made a lot easier by giving some advance thought to how you will approach the event.

If you're new to the distance and your priority is to get round, it helps to break it down into three lots of four miles, four lots of three miles or even six lots of two miles. Followed by a mile and a little bit at the end. It's much more manageable to tackle these distances in your head and to gauge how you feel and how to pace the next section of the race than to continually have the idea of 13 miles of running playing over and over through your mind.

Decide in advance how you are going to fuel and hydrate

yourself during the race and whether or not this plan makes use of the water/drink stations along the route or if you are taking your own supplies. Bringing your own food and drink means that you can eat or drink what you are used to during the race. You can also break up the event with refuelling while having total control over your schedule, which you often don't have if you rely on the race organisers. After all, you may wish to refuel more regularly than they think is necessary.

EVERYBODY NEEDS GOOD NEIGHBOURS

During the race, it helps to keep an eye on those around you. Pick out some people running at the same pace as you and use them as a guide, to help you maintain your pace throughout the race. Remember, it's fine to change "pacer" during a race if you need to speed up or slow down. It's just useful to keep your eye on someone rather than feeling that you're doing all the work alone.

If you're a seasoned half-marathon runner and you're looking for a PB, you'll need to approach the day slightly differently. You should have a very clear idea of your target finishing time and also your target-mile split times. Use the week before the race to take a really good look at the course and plan how you will pace yourself. Look in particular at the course profile and see exactly where you might lose speed going uphill and where you might gain it back again heading down the other side. You need to factor this into your split times so you're not too surprised if it looks like you are ahead of or behind schedule at any given mile marker.

In addition to watching your split times, you also need to monitor how you feel continuously and react appropriately. It's likely that with the excitement of the day and a rush of adrenalin, you'll feel great for the first couple of miles. Resist the temptation to gain some time here and stay on schedule. If you go out too fast, your PB won't happen. If you still feel great further into the race then it's fine to hit the gas a bit. Any point from mile ten onwards is a good time to begin stretching your legs a little bit, but make any rise in speed a very gradual one as you make your way over the last two to three miles.

❝ *Pick out some people running at the same pace as you and use them as a guide.* **❞**

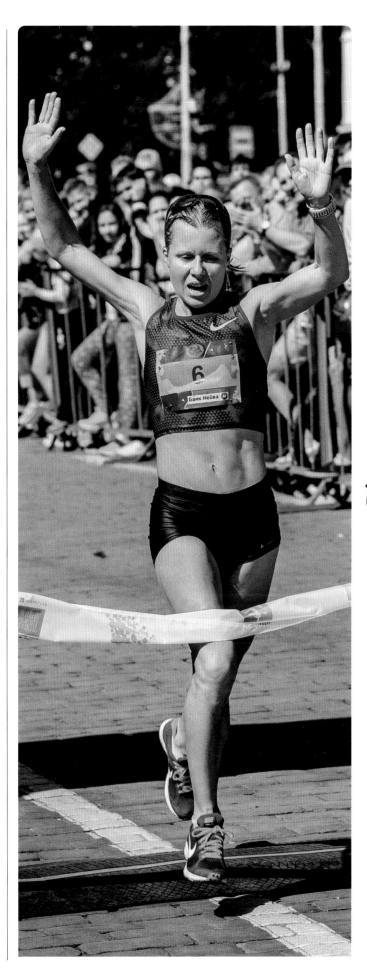

MARATHON TIPS

From discovering different surfaces to tackling the dreaded "wall", this is where one of the most daunting distances is at last demystified.

Most of us are creatures of habit, following the same few routes when we run. Perhaps it's three laps of the park, the usual river path or a circuit around the houses. Whatever the surface, if you run on it often, it will have a powerful impact on your body and if you're not fit, that impact could be a negative one. "Training on different surfaces if you're doing a marathon is not essential, but it can reduce the impact on your joints," says personal trainer and marathon runner Anne-Marie Lategan. 'For experienced runners, I would recommend a variety of surfaces because you know your running style and will know how to adapt to different surfaces. But for beginners, I would say practise on the surface that matches your race."

Peta Bee, runner and fitness author, says: "I believe your muscles and ligaments should be tested in a variety of ways; changing terrain forces you to adapt your running speed accordingly. My old coach used to get us running up log steps in nearby woods instead of doing gym work once a week. Of course, the majority of your training runs should be on the road or trails, but by adding at least two different types of training a week, the roads will suddenly seem a lot easier."

STRONG MUSCLES
Well-exercised muscles do their job – contracting and lengthening as you run to offload the impact of your feet hitting the ground when you run. With each foot-strike your body is subject to impact forces that amount to several times your weight. This impact travels into the foot, then the knee, then to the hip, then the lower back and so on; if problems occur, it will be in the weakest area. In general, roads or pavements are the worst surfaces to run on. But each type of terrain affects the body in a different way and your individual weak spots and fitness levels will respond accordingly. For example, uneven off-road conditions can be problematic for anyone with poor stabilising muscles and weak ankles. Protect yourself by wearing the right shoes. Some trainers absorb a huge amount of impact from the ground; others offer less protection. Choose what feels right, not what looks best.

> *" If you're doing a marathon, training on different surfaces is not essential but it can reduce the impact on your joints. "*

RUNNING SURFACES EXPLAINED

CONCRETE
This is the harshest surface to run on because there's no "give" as you land. If you're going on a long training run, try to do some of your run on a grass verge to minimise the impact, or build in a route around a park.

TREADMILL
Provides a reasonable amount of cushioning from the high-impact nature of running, so it's worth using it once a week. Avoid too much, though: remember, you need to get your body used to the elements for race day.

GRASS
Is one of the best surfaces to run on, because it will provide some cushioning and it certainly has less impact on your joints than concrete does. Just be careful not to run in long grass, where you won't see any dips or uneven terrain that could lead to injury.

TRAIL/OFF-ROAD
Can be ideal for varying the impact through the joints and ligaments, but make sure you run in well-lit areas and be careful you don't twist an ankle or hurt your knees. You will be putting more pressure on your lower body, which will have to work harder to stabilise you and keep you balanced.

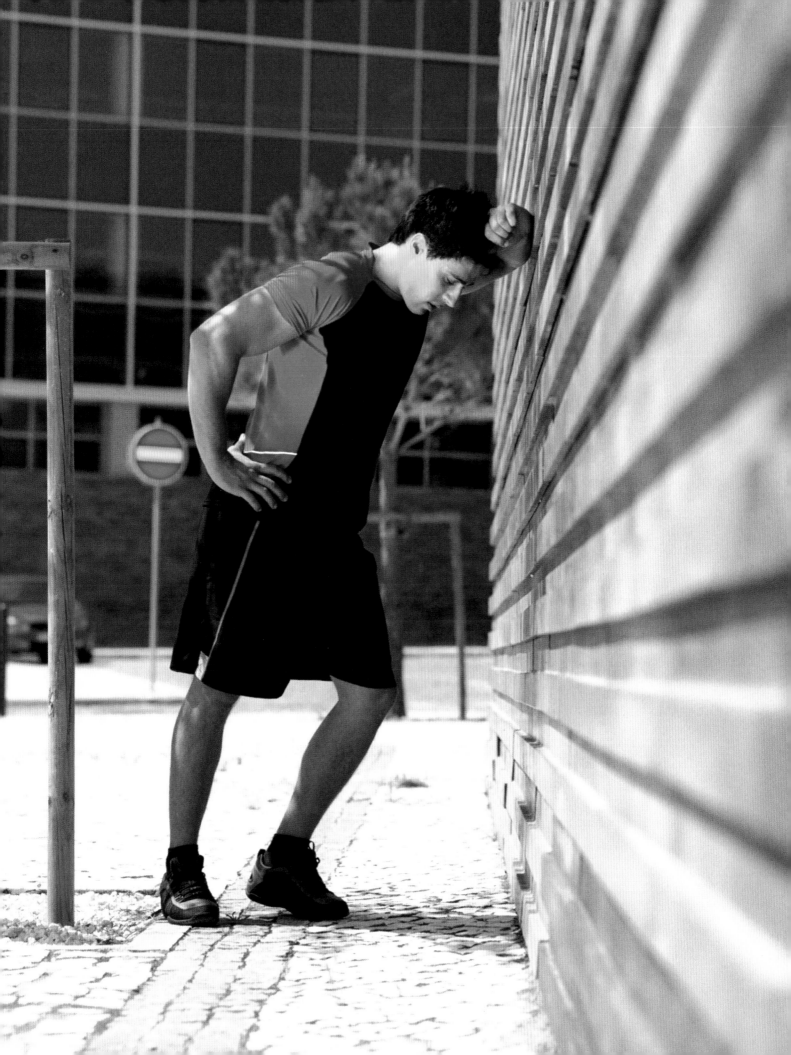

AVOID THE WALL

Reduce your training by 30 per cent two weeks before your marathon, just jogging and doing a few sprints in the week before the race. This is will ensure your body can rest, recover and become saturated with carbs.
Regularly practise your long run.
Don't start the race too fast. If you do, you may feel terrific in the first three miles but the chances are that you'll crash and burn before the end of the race.

TEAR DOWN THE WALL

If you've ever watched television coverage of a marathon, you'll have seen the jelly-legged runners staggering towards the finish line looking like they are carrying a bus on their back. They've hit the "wall". You don't really know what it is until you hit it and then you never forget it – your legs go on strike and a full body insurrection takes place, usually around mile 20 of the 26.2-mile race. It's as blunt and immovable a barricade as it sounds. You feel stuck where you are. There's just no way around or over it. You crash into it and through it, to emerge in a crumpled heap on the other side.

BACK UP THE CARBS

Some experts say it's not willpower the afflicted lack, but carbs. Humans simply weren't designed to go the long haul without sustenance. Carbohydrates are stored as glycogen in the muscles and liver, but even a full tank will run out after 60 to 90 minutes of intense exercise. Novice and ill-prepared runners often try to go the distance on too few carbohydrate calories, which can be their downfall. "Maintaining a diet containing 60 to 70 per cent carbohydrates in the days before an endurance event will ensure you start the race with high muscle-glycogen stores," says Louise Sutton, dietician at the Carnegie Centre for Sports Performance at Leeds Metropolitan University "Topping up energy reserves with isotonic carbohydrate drinks from the start is also a useful preventative tactic." She adds that, as with the

"Topping up energy reserves with isotonic carbohydrate drinks from the start is also a useful preventative tactic."

EAT TO RUN

CARB-LOADING

A week-long regime involving an exhaustive bout of running followed by a carbohydrate-depletion diet and three days of high-carb intake – was popular in the 1970s and 1980s but has been proven to be detrimental. Instead, aim to consume 60 to 70 per cent of your daily calorie intake as carbs, maintaining this ratio in the three days before the race.

BREAD AND PASTA

Low-fat carbohydrate foods, but also aim to increase your intake of low-GI carbs, which deliver the longest-lasting energy boost. Try bananas, apples, tinned peaches or – Paula Radcliffe's choice before a marathon – porridge.

INCLUDE SOME LOW-FAT PROTEIN

Such as yoghurt and eggs in your daily diet – endurance athletes burn it, as well as carbs, for energy.

CONSUME 30 TO 60 GRAMS OF CARBOHYDRATE EVERY HOUR

As recommended by the American College of Sports Medicine. That's the equivalent of 120 to 240 calories. As little as 50 grams of carbohydrate can bring your brain and body back to normal in 10 to 15 minutes. Isotonic sports drinks provide the optimum ratio of carbohydrate, fluid and electrolytes (or body salts). Some runners prefer to keep a stock of jelly beans or barley sugars in their pocket.

half-marathon (see pp. 78–9) staying well hydrated is important too. "Being even a little dehydrated slows gastric emptying – the removal of food from your gut into your bloodstream. That means your body finds it harder to obtain carbohydrate as fuel."

Diet isn't the only preventative measure. Making sure your body is physically and nutritionally primed is crucial. Attending to race-day practicalities, again focusing on your diet, can also make a crucial difference. "If it's an early start, your last major meal should be the evening before, but don't make it so big that it sits uncomfortably the next day," says Sutton. "Eat breakfast, but nothing you haven't tried before."

KNOW YOUR DRINK STATIONS

Check when, where or even if isotonic drinks will be distributed along the course. If sports drinks are supplied, find out which brand will be available, train with it to check it agrees with you. If not, bring your tried and trusted brand to keep your carb levels topped up during the race.

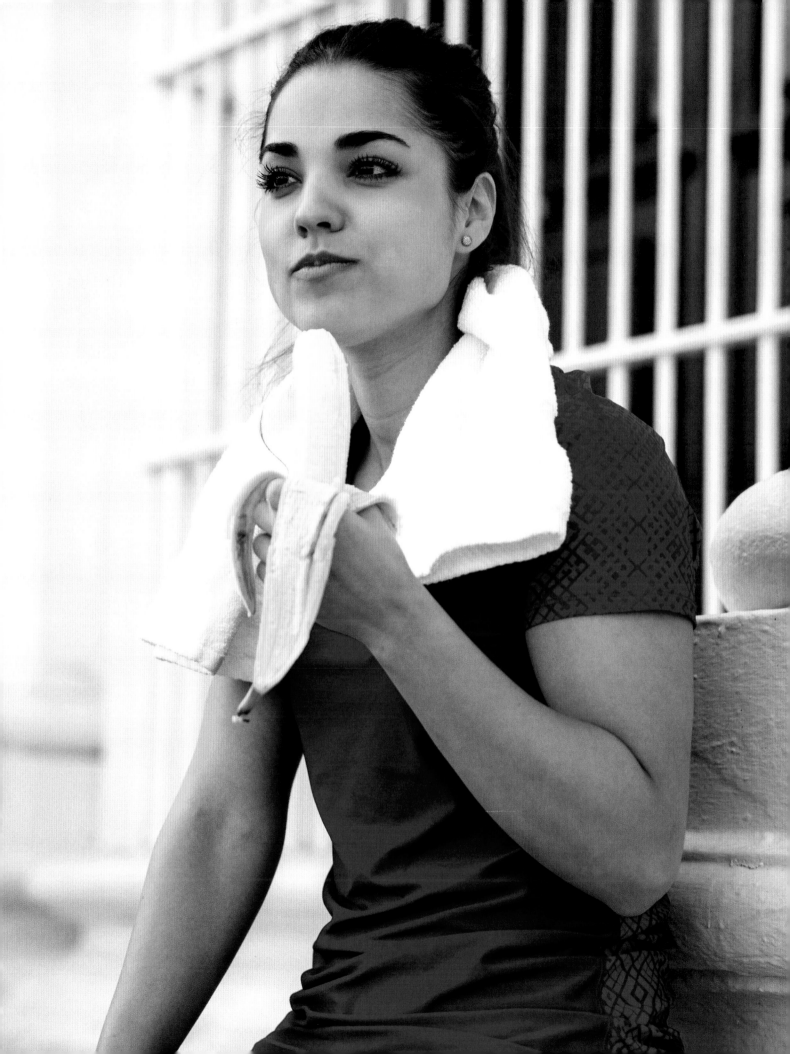

ELITE MARATHON SECRETS

You might never run a sub-2-hour 30-minute marathon or blast out a 30-minute 10K on the track, but there's plenty you can learn from those who do.

We can never be like the elite runners, the Olympic medal-winners. But we can learn something from their training methods.

ALTITUDE TENTS

These are sealed see-through tents that athletes sleep in. Living or training at altitude causes the body to adapt to the lower oxygen content by producing more oxygen-carrying red blood cells and haemoglobin. This will provide enhanced performance when returning to a lower altitude. They may cost you about £4,000; however, you can hire then from about £60 per week. "It was very beneficial prior to going to altitude training as I seemed to hit the ground running once I arrived at the camp," said Olympian Jenny Meadows, who has won World and European Championship medals. "I also found that when I returned from altitude training the benefits lasted longer through continued use of the tent." It's recommended that you get up to 12–14 hours' exposure per day. "I found that this was unrealistic so wasn't sure if I was benefitting as much as I hoped. Since I stopped using the tent I am sleeping much better."

ZERO GRAVITY TREADMILL

Developed originally for astronauts, expect to run with your legs in a "bubble" that uses air pressure to gently lift you as you run. Brad Neal, a specialist musculoskeletal physiotherapist says any runner can benefit from the Alter G treadmill. "They are especially useful when recovering from a stress fracture or medial tibial stress syndrome (shin splints)." Alter G sessions in a centre can cost as little as £20-30.

CHANGE THE RULES: 80/20

Exercise physiologist Stephen Seiler, from the University of Adger, Norway, created the 80/20 rule – where 80 per cent of your workouts should be done at a slow speed, coupled with 20 per cent at a medium-to-fast pace, for maximum performance gains. "Elite athletes don't train as hard as they can every session," Seiler said. "They can't. You shouldn't either." He also believes elites will choose to hold back the last few per cent on intensity in order to be able to accumulate more minutes. "This might mean doing 8 x 1 minute intervals at 90 per cent HR [heart rate] max instead of 3 x 1 minute intervals at 94 per cent." A tiny decrease in intensity translates to a large increase in accumulated work time. Don't let the easy sessions become harder in search of a little extra - a classic training error.

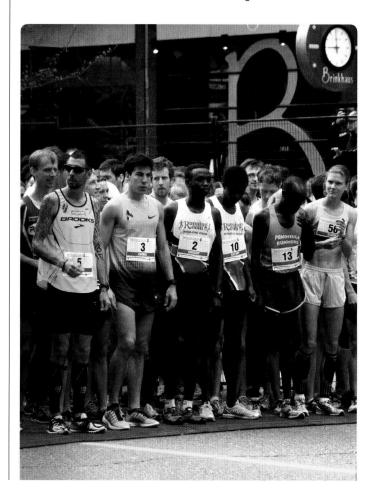

PLAN TO PEAK

"Plan training to ensure that you will be at your absolute best for your target race," said London marathon runner Amy Whitehead. "Work backwards from race day and outline the sessions/races that you wish to complete to give you the confidence that you can achieve your goal. For a marathon, a 12-14 week build up is ideal. Have the confidence to know when the training is banked. Resist the urge to complete one last hard training session. This mental discipline is really challenging, but essential to ensure that you are genuinely more refreshed and truly ready to rock on race day. There is a reason why Bolt looks so chilled out before race day!"

MENTAL TRAINING

"In training I would practise mental tricks I might use in a race," said UK marathon runner Mara Yamauchi, "such as setting myself small goals, focusing on my arm action, telling myself I was running well and so on."

FARTLEK

"This was one of my favourite sessions," said Jenny Meadows. "I would usually do this for 20-30 minutes. I would do a five-minute jog followed by ten minutes of 20 seconds of faster effort with 40 seconds easy jog recovery between and then five minutes of easy jogging to cool down. You get 10 x 20 seconds of good paced running and your heart rate is really high for the whole ten-minute work section. The duration, pace and interval lengths change depending on each runner."

> *" Mental discipline is really challenging, but essential to ensure that you are genuinely more refreshed and truly ready to rock on race day. "*

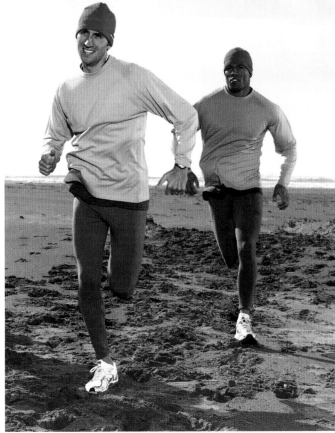

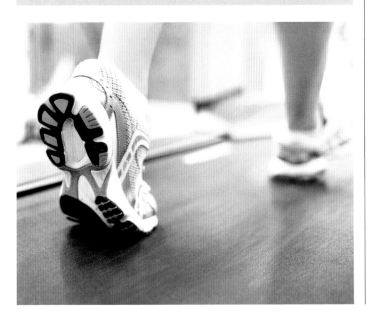

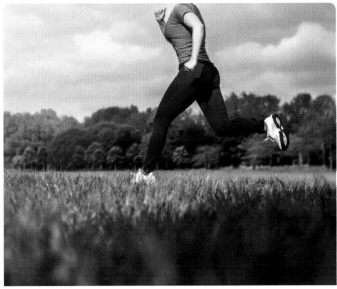

ULTRA-MARATHON AND ENDURANCE TIPS

After you've done your marathon, you may want to follow it up with another goal. So maybe, just maybe, an ultra-marathon is the way to go.

Completing a marathon is an extraordinary achievement and let no one tell you otherwise. And once you've done one, the chances are good that you'll do another, then another. And one day you may begin to think about longer distances; you may find your attention turning to an ultra-marathon.

Many of us shy away from ultras because we erroneously believe that to do an ultra you have to be ultra-fast or ultra-hard. But you simply have to want to do one, believe you can do one (many experts say that up to 80 per cent of ultra-success comes from mental strength) and willing to put in the training.

An "ultra" is anything longer than a marathon. So if you had a long walk to the station after a completing a marathon, you've already done an ultra of sorts. The different race lengths mean that you could start with 30 miles, fewer than four miles longer than a marathon. Many ultras are multi-stage events so you don't have to complete the entire distance in one day and can fully enjoy the unique camaraderie of an ultra at the end of a stage.

MORE MILES

If you enjoyed your marathon training, the extra distance you'll have to now put in need not take over your life. "If you're targeting a 40-, 50- or 60-miler then you need to have a solid marathon base and simply add several weeks of decent long runs," said personal trainer and ultra-runner Ian Campbell. "I favour the three-weeks-hard/one-week-easy training pattern to give your body time to recover. Aim to do one long, easy run of four to six hours combined with perhaps one or two semi-long runs (over ten miles) per week plus speed work and threshold runs to keep up the momentum."

The rule of thumb is that the longer the distance, the longer the training period you need, so for the 56-mile Comrades Marathon in South Africa, Don Oliver, former Comrades Marathon coach and author, has suggested a 21-week programme during which you run between 5K and 12K five days a week and then do a longer run – anything from 15K to, eventually, 65K – on Sundays.

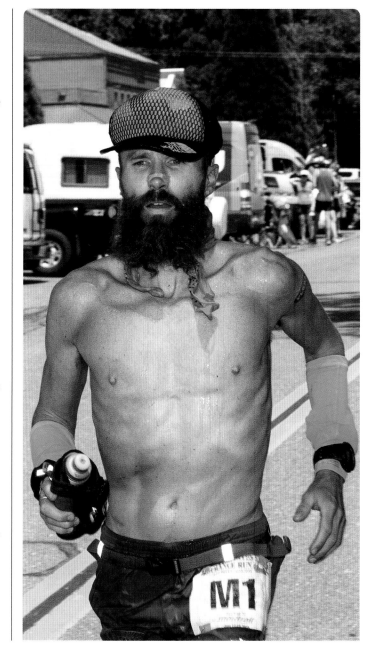

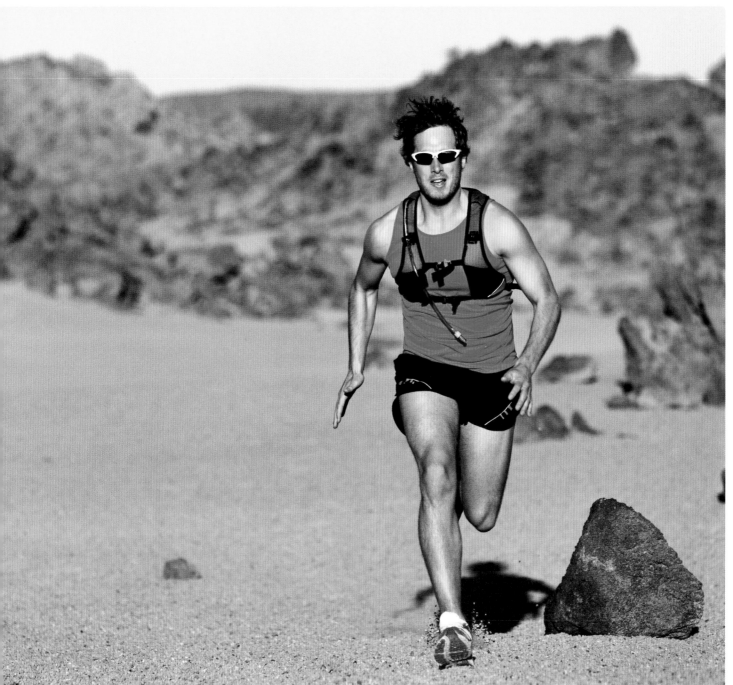

THE MENTAL RACE

According to Campbell, no matter what your body type, if you have completed a marathon you are capable of doing an ultra-marathon. Oliver also said, "Comrades runners come in all shapes and sizes but what really matters is having a strong mind. Training always improves your body's performance but the most important benefit that results from those long hours on the road is the development of stamina and perseverance."

It's also interesting to note that if you're a slow marathon runner you'll have an advantage over faster runners simply because you'll already be used to spending far more time on your feet. You'll probably also be familiar with taking walk breaks, which, for anyone

bar elite ultra-marathoners, are normal. Campbell said: "It's advisable to incorporate power-walking breaks into your training so that you're familiar with them before the race. Use them to practise eating and drinking. If your target ultra is much longer than 30 miles you generally won't be able to survive on gels and water alone, so get used to carrying your provisions in a backpack or belt and eating while you're running. Try bananas, sports bars, salty biscuits and chocolate, plus gels, and see what suits you." Above all, don't leave anything to chance. Find out beforehand what will be on offer at the aid stations, and experiment as much as possible in your training so that there are no surprises on the day.

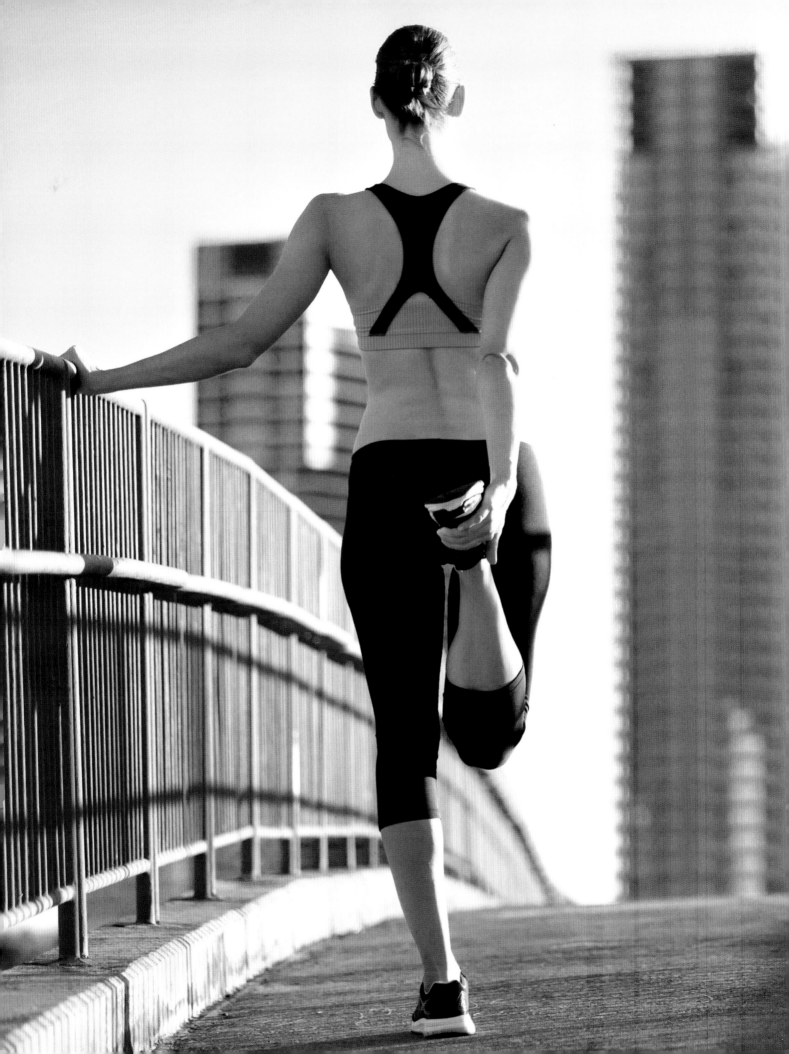

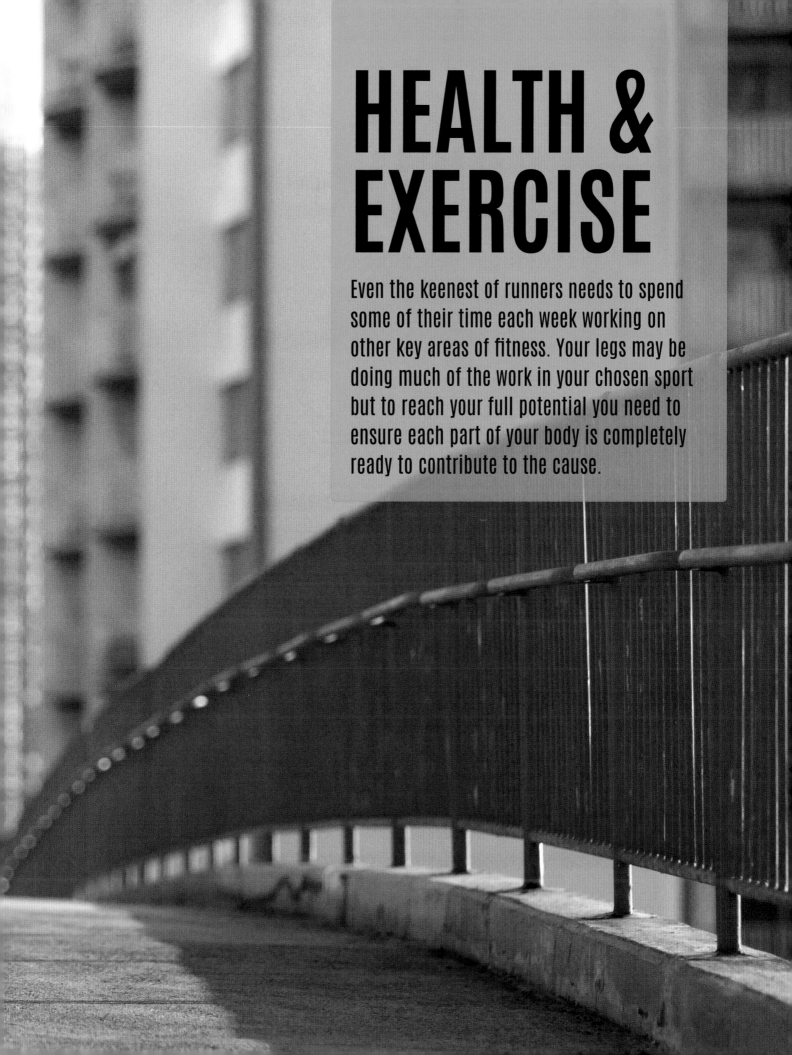

HEALTH & EXERCISE

Even the keenest of runners needs to spend some of their time each week working on other key areas of fitness. Your legs may be doing much of the work in your chosen sport but to reach your full potential you need to ensure each part of your body is completely ready to contribute to the cause.

THE IMPORTANCE OF EXERCISING

An in-depth look at the whole-body fitness approach.

If you're doing three running sessions a week, use another two to work on strength and conditioning. When we run, a force equal to approximately three times our bodyweight goes through the knees. It can improve bone density but you need to build up your strength. Stronger muscles are less likely to suffer from strains, pulls or tears.

Good upper-body strength will benefit you as it means your arms will be able to pump more powerfully, especially during the latter stages of a race where you may want to run faster. And a strong back will help you maintain good posture while you run. Foot strength is important for running, as it's the first part of the body to absorb the impact. However, many of us don't even think about it. Gripping exercises for the feet can help. Try to wiggle your toes separately, or put one foot on a piece of paper and try to scrunch it up. There are also gym and non-running sessions that look at other aspects of your fitness.

90

GLUTE STRENGTH

HILL WALKING
Either up a steep hill or incline walking on the treadmill. This targets your glute strength. You make a big hip extension movement during running and if it doesn't come from the glutes, the only other option for the body is to take on that loading and force. And that loads other muscles, like hamstrings. Tight hamstrings can often lead to other issues such as knee problems.
WATCH OUT FOR - poor posture. Keep your shoulders up and chest lifted.

KETTLEBELL CLASSES
improve total-body strength, core and leg power. The kettlebell swing also engages the hamstrings and glutes.
WATCH OUT FOR - poor technique. The kettlebell swing should be a hinge from the hips, not a squat.

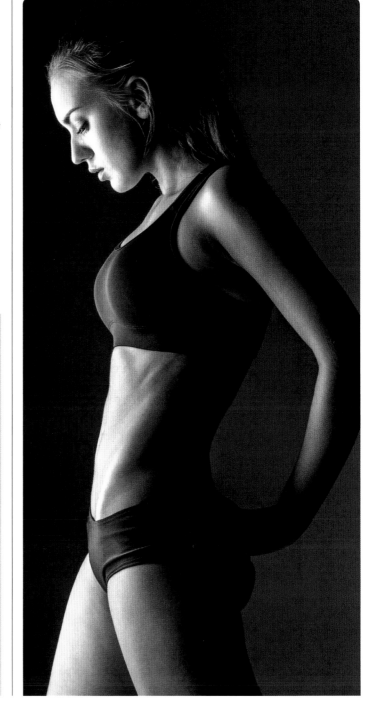

STRONG THIGHS AND HAMSTRINGS

SPIN CLASSES

During hill climbs you'll work the quadriceps hard and during standing sprints you'll also feel your hamstrings and glutes working. Good for hamstring endurance.

WATCH OUT FOR – having the seat the wrong height as this can cause knee pain. The seat should be level with your hip when you're standing next to the bike.

ALL-OVER ENDURANCE AND STAMINA

CIRCUIT TRAINING

Which is moving from one workstation to another without a break, which will improve your cardiovascular fitness and also your muscular endurance, as you'll be doing strength exercises like push-ups, mountain climbers and squats.

WATCH OUT FOR – poor exercise technique as you get tired.

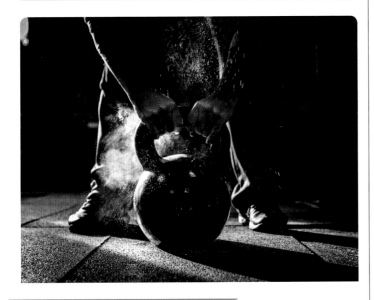

ACCELERATION

RACQUET SPORTS

In which the sudden, fast explosive movements as you sprint to reach the ball or shuttlecock can mean you'll feel the benefit in a crowded race.

WATCH OUT FOR – too much impact. Be careful about not overdoing it and avoid playing squash the day after a hard run, when your body is still recovering. Warm up thoroughly before you start playing and have a proper stretch afterwards.

CORE STRENGTH

DYNAMIC CORE EXERCISES

Instead of doing a normal plank or side plank, which don't involve any movement. Look at mountain climbers or squat thrusts, because they get you moving just as running does.

WATCH OUT FOR – poor technique. Try to keep your core tight. Rest when you need to. Mountain climber and squat thrusts are hard.

UPPER-BODY STRENGTH

CABLE EXERCISES

For when you run and your arms go back and forth.

WATCH OUT FOR – poor technique. Cables can be confusing if you've not used them before, so ask a gym instructor to show you how to set them up.

SWIMMING

Is particularly good for the shoulders and upper back. If you swim with a pull buoy you can focus solely on upper body and give your legs a rest.

WATCH OUT FOR – poor technique. Avoid breaststroke if you have knee issues, as when the legs extend and are then brought back together the knee rotates outwards. As a hinge joint, the knee is designed to move back and forward, not outwards, so the inner ligament of the knee can be put under strain.

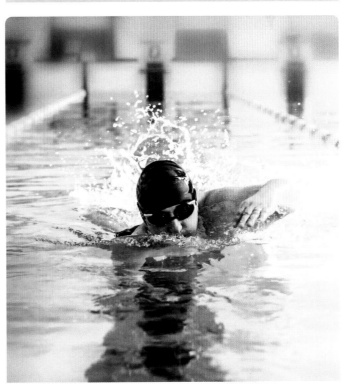

COMMON INJURIES AND HOW TO AVOID THEM

With an increase in training volume comes an increased risk of getting injured. Here's how to lower your chances of coming a cropper.

When you're training for longer distances, there's a good chance you're going to develop a niggling pain at some point and if you're unlucky this can turn into an injury. This goes for first-timers as well as experienced runners: it comes with the territory. However, it's more likely to happen when you increase your mileage, and therefore the chance and form of overuse injuries. This is not so surprising when you consider the forces and punishing impact involved in running.

In one hour, you may take 4–5,000 strides on each leg and the force travels through the whole body from the heel. Your knee joints absorb and dissipate a large percentage of the force from the ground and your thighs absorb about 60 per cent of the force, reducing further stresses to joints. As you get tired, you can't absorb the force as well and the repetitive loading can cause injury. But with good preparation and technique, you can train injury-free and enjoy your running.

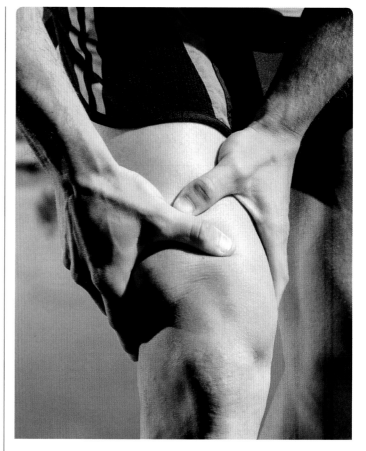

RUNNER'S KNEE

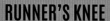

DIAGNOSIS
Pain around the kneecap or patella, also known as patellofemoral pain. Injuries include chondromalacia patellae, which is damage to cartilage at the back of the kneecap.

CAUSE
Many factors: increased loading and frequency of running, weakness in the thigh muscles, muscular imbalances, tightness of the iliotibial band (ITB), poor lower-limb stability or increased foot pronation.

PREVENTION
Maintain quad strength, flexibility and lower-limb stability.

HEALING
A few weeks up to a few months, depending on cause and severity.

> *"In one hour, you may take 4-5,000 strides on each leg and the force travels through the whole body from the heel."*

STRESS FRACTURE

DIAGNOSIS
A micro-fracture in bone that occurs from repetitive loading. It usually occurs in the lower leg or small bones of the foot, but can also affect the thigh bone.

CAUSE
Increasing the loading on the legs too quickly. Bone remodels when extra demands are placed on it – when you load and stress your bone, it gradually becomes stronger. However, when you load too fast, the remodelling of the bone tissue cannot occur quickly enough to compensate for the stress.

PREVENTION
Don't increase the intensity or duration of your runs too quickly and have rest days. If you have pain, don't run – get examined.

HEALING
Six to eight weeks.

SHIN SPLINTS

DIAGNOSIS
The days when any type of pain in the shin area was labelled "shin splints" are long gone. Sports physiotherapists, doctors or podiatrists will tell you that the pain might be coming from repetitive strain to the shin bone (tibia), which may lead to a stress fracture if severe. But it may also be coming from tight calf muscles, irritation to the connective tissue around the calf muscles, trapped nerves or aggravated tendons... the list goes on. It is worth getting a sports medicine professional to assess you properly. Most shin problems are caused by the repeated impact involved in running. Without adequate rest and recovery time, the bone, muscle and tendon can become irritated and start to lose strength.

CAUSE
Increasing duration or intensity quickly is a common cause, and poor footwear and over-pronation are biomechanical influences. Metabolic bone health (reduced bone density) may contribute too.

PREVENTION
By increasing intensity and duration gradually, stretching your calves regularly and making sure you're wearing appropriate footwear.

HEALING
Takes up to six weeks, depending on severity.

PREVENTION

- Perform a dynamic warm-up, including running with high knees, mini jumps and running while kicking your heels up to your bottom.
- Wear correct footwear.
- Pay attention to nutrition and hydration. Follow a well-planned schedule.
- Improve your leg strength, stability and balance.
- Have at least one complete rest day each week.
- Incorporate low-impact cross training, such as cycling or swimming, into your training.
- Consult a physio if you feel any pain.

EXERCISES TO PREVENT INJURY

You can employ some simple exercises to become strong in the right areas and significantly reduce your chance of picking up an injury. And if you are unlucky enough to develop a niggle, you'll be strong enough to quickly bounce back. Make them part of your everyday routine to strengthen the kinetic chain used when running. You will strengthen and lengthen everything at breakfast to help your knee, the most common area of injury for runners. Then exercise and stretch your calves at lunchtime to reduce Achilles' and heel pain and work the sides of your thighs for greater control on those long training runs. Keeping these exercises simple means you're more likely to fit them into your daily routine. Make a little effort and you'll notice a lot of improvement.

93

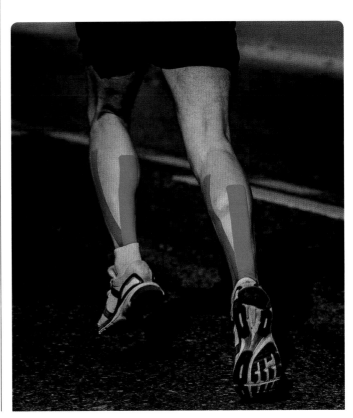

THE BREAKFAST ROUTINE

- Stand on one leg and balance for 20 to 30 seconds before changing sides. This improves your proprioception (balance and spatial awareness), as well as developing functional strength in your ankles, knees, hips and core.

- Walk sideways along your hallway, ideally with a loop of exercise band around your thighs, strengthening your inner and outer thighs (abductors and adductors). This can be made more difficult if you try to carry the morning cup of tea back to your bedroom at the same time.

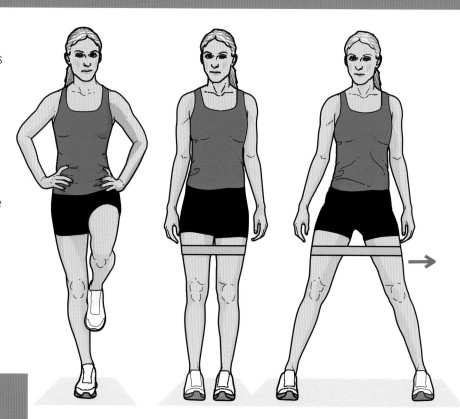

94

THE LUNCH ROUTINE

- Find a stairwell at work and use the bottom step to work your calf muscles. First, stand on tiptoes on the bottom step and then slowly lower yourself down until your heel is at the lowest point; remain there for a few seconds to stretch, then return back up at a normal pace, before slowly lowering again. Do three sets of 15 reps on each leg.

- Stretch the muscles that operate your ITB by placing one foot around the back of the other until your little toes are touching, then lean to the side (if the right foot goes around the back, then lean to the left, and vice versa). Adapt this stretch by now leaning forwards and twisting to the side.

- Strengthen your knee control with the single-leg squat. This exercise is the greatest pre-training tool for those beginning a marathon journey. Standing on one leg, bend your knee just enough so that it would be visible through a pair of leggings and then straighten. Repeat this hundreds of times a day for two weeks, then progress to a knee bend that lowers your hip about two inches for a further two weeks.

- Continue to develop every fortnight, until you have a controlled knee bend of 65-80 degrees. This will ensure the slow progress and development of key muscles in your foot, knee and hip, which becomes transferable to your running technique and reduces your risk of injury.

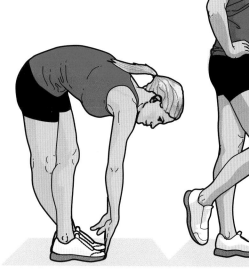

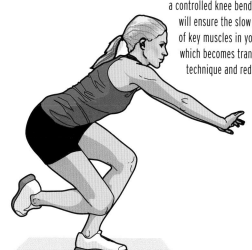

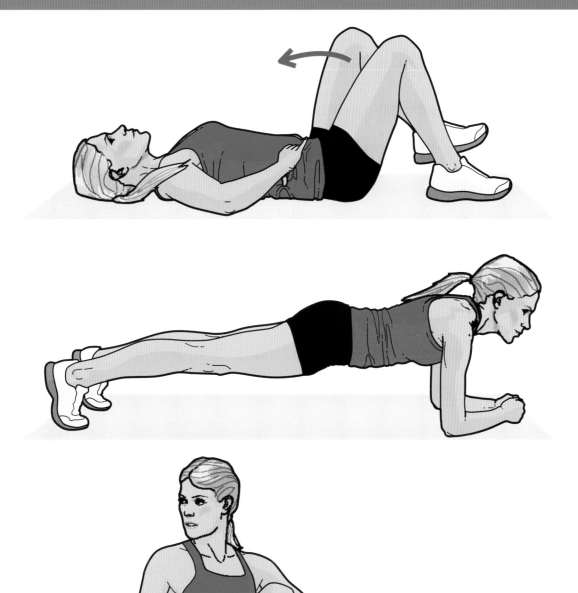

THE DINNER ROUTINE

- Lie on the floor, knees bent and feet flat. Tighten the muscles in your lower stomach and draw your belly button in towards your spine. Keeping everything tight, slowly lift each foot six inches off the ground in turn. Do three sets of 25 reps with each foot.

- Enter a press-up position and then place your forearms on the ground with your elbows aligned below the shoulders, and arms parallel to your body. Clasp your hands beneath your head and hold the position for as long as possible. This is great for your core strength.

- Stretch your glutes by sitting down with a straight back. Cross one leg over the other and pull the knee towards the opposite shoulder, while twisting towards your crossed knee. Hold for 20 seconds and swap sides. Stretch each glute five times.

MANAGING INJURIES

Be aware of all aspects of your running body and take care to prevent problems where you can before they arise.

Talk to any runner about injuries they most want to avoid, and you're likely to be met with a variety of painful-sounding ailments. Most leg and lower back problems feature high up on the worry list. And don't neglect your feet until it's too late and something goes wrong, as runners often do.

FEET

BLISTERS
CAUSE
Heat and friction, when your trainers or socks rub your feet.
TREATMENT
If the blister is small and unbroken, protect it with a specialist blister plaster. Drain larger blisters by piercing with a sterilised needle and applying antibiotic cream.
PREVENTION
Correctly fitting shoes and specialist socks that regulate temperature.

BLACK TOENAILS
CAUSE
Toes repeatedly come into contact with your shoes.
TREATMENT
Soaking feet in warm, salty water.
PREVENTION
Buy running shoes that are half a size bigger than your normal size so your feet can expand with heat.

ACHILLES TENDINOPATHY
CAUSE
Pain in the Achilles tendon is most often caused by tight calf muscles, over-pronation or a sudden increase in training.
TREATMENT
This shouldn't be left untreated, in case the tendon ruptures. Stretch tight calf muscles using slow lowering exercises, called eccentric exercises, where you concentrate on lowering your heel over the edge of a step.
PREVENTION
Correct shoes and get orthotics if need be.

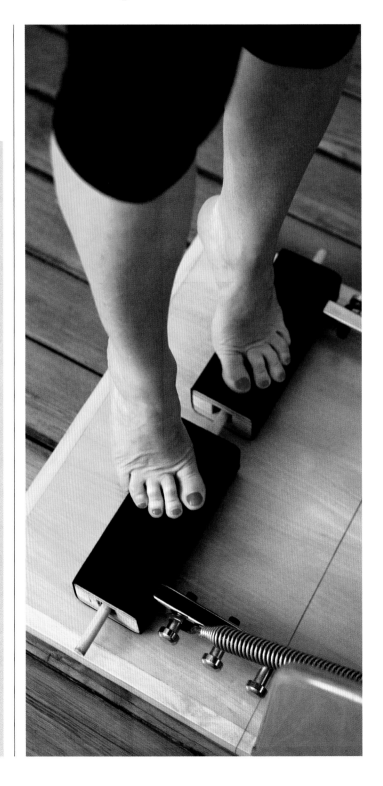

BACK FOR GOOD

If you have recently hurt your back and are returning to running after a period of rest, you may experience pain in your back due to impact. It is your back telling you that it is not quite ready for running yet. Spend more time working on your core stability muscles and doing non-impact cardiovascular work.

Most running injuries involve the foot, shins and knee, but the forces can sometimes be transmitted further up to the hip, pelvis and low back. Your running biomechanics can also play a part if you have a malalignment, particularly around the hips and pelvis. This can be a problem for people who have one leg longer than the other or an imbalance in the muscles causing asymmetry. The pain can be transmitted to the lower back and also to other areas such as the hamstring, the leg and the foot. This type of back pain tends to start a short while into the run, gradually worsens, but disappears soon after you stop. Most alignment problems need to be assessed by a biomechanical specialist.

HAMMING IT UP

Endurance runners are less likely to suffer from hamstring strains than sprinters. However, if there is poor movement control around the pelvis and core, you can sometimes get irritation where the hamstrings attach, either up in the buttock or down by the knee.

Weak hamstrings can also affect the control of movement of the knee, which can contribute to injuries such as patella-tracking problems, or iliotibial band friction syndrome (ITBFS). Runners who have lower hamstring strength in one leg are more likely to suffer from a hamstring-related injury. Problems are likely to occur after an inadequate warm-up or towards the end of a running session when muscles are more fatigued.

Warm up before any running session. Remember that endurance running works your quadriceps more than your hamstrings, which can create a strength imbalance. Work through some strengthening exercises. Strong gluteal muscles can take the load off the hamstrings. Work on core stability and balance because this can improve the control of movement around the pelvis, making your running more efficient.

If your day is sedentary, your hamstrings can gradually become short and tight. Gently stretching out the hamstrings for 30 seconds or longer each day can help. There are mixed views as to whether hamstring flexibility reduces the risk of injury, but it is generally accepted that people with tight muscles are more likely to strain them. If you have good hamstring length, you should be able to sit on the floor with your bottom all the way back against a wall with your knees straight. The biggest risk factor for hamstring injury is having had a previous hamstring injury. If so, you will need to address all the factors above.

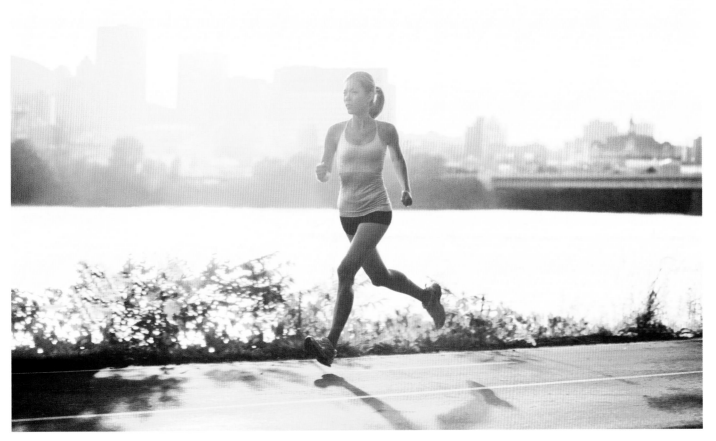

PRE-RUN STRETCHING AND EXERCISING

To avoid injury and also improve the quality of your runs you must warm up before you take off. Easy mobilisation exercises can help you along the way.

STANDING GLUTE LIFTS

Good activation of your glutes during your run will stabilise your hips and prevent back and knee problems.

TECHNIQUE
- Stand on your right leg and lean slightly forwards from your waist.
- Hold on to a secure object to aid your balance.
- Bend your left knee and flex your foot (pull your toes up).
- Push your left leg back and up.
- Slowly lower with control.
- Complete ten repetitions on the right before changing over to the left.

Warming up before a run helps prepare your body for the task ahead. It will increase the oxygen delivery to the muscles and make your muscles more pliable. Many people do static stretches before a run, but research has shown these are of little value at this point and may even have a negative impact on your performance. However, mobilising exercises can improve your workout.

Mobilisation means moving your muscles and joints to increase blood supply to warm up the muscles and fluid in joints. Lubricating your joints before a run will improve your performance and highlight any niggling pains. Mobilisation exercises differ from stretching because they are slow, controlled movements throughout a specific range of motion, whereas stretching lengthens muscles and can cause micro-tears, which can be made worse during a long run. Before you run, make sure you walk for at least five minutes, so you raise your heart rate gradually. This will help reduce the risk of injuries or minor niggles due to cold muscles.

MULTI-DIRECTIONAL LUNGES

Running on uneven surfaces puts your ankles, knees and hips under constant pressure to adapt. The better your mobilisation during your warm-up, the better you'll cope with changes in running surfaces.

TECHNIQUE
- Stand with your feet comfortably apart.
- Step forwards with your right leg and bend both legs to perform a lunge.
- Step back to the starting position and lunge sideways.
- Return to the starting position once more and lunge backwards.
- Complete one set on the right before changing over to the left.
- Do five multi-directional lunges per side.

HIP SWINGS

Hip swings improve the movement around your hips and ensure sufficient shock absorption.

TECHNIQUE
- Stand in front of a wall or fence and place your hands on it a shoulder-width apart.
- Lean slightly forwards from your hips.
- Swing your right leg in front of you from side to side.
- Complete one set of ten repetitions before changing over to the left leg.

SPINE ROTATIONS

Your spine acts as a shock absorber, so it's important to mobilise it during your warm-up.

TECHNIQUE
• Sit on the floor with your legs wide apart.
• Lean with both hands towards your right foot.
• Slowly walk your hands over to the middle and then to the left foot, while stretching as far forward as possible.
• Return to the starting position.
• Reverse the move back to your right foot.
• Do five to ten rotations.

SHOULDER ROTATIONS

Your arm swing plays an important role in regulating your speed, so it's important to increase the mobility of your shoulder joints

TECHNIQUE
• Stand with your feet a shoulder-width apart and your arms extended out to the sides.
• Rotate your arms ten times forwards and backwards.
• Make the circles as big as possible. changing over to the left leg.

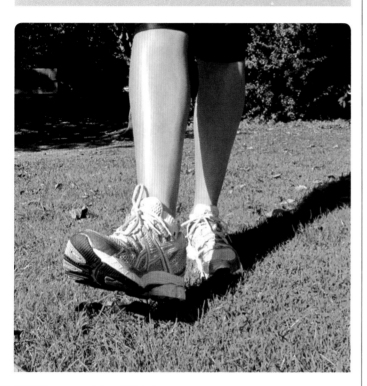

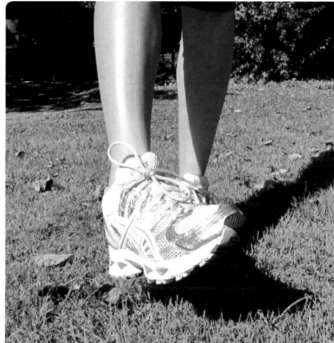

ANKLE ROTATIONS

Your feet and ankles control the first point of contact with the ground, so it's important to ensure they are warmed up to prevent twisting or straining this complex mechanism.

TECHNIQUE
• Stand on your right leg while rotating your left ankle in a clockwise direction.
• Ensure you pull your toes up and point as much as you can.
• Complete one set of ten repetitions before changing to an anti-clockwise direction.
Repeat on the right ankle.

" Mobilisation exercises are slow, controlled movements, whereas stretching lengthens muscles. "

POST-RUN STRETCHING AND EXERCISING

Whether you have just a few minutes or over an hour to invest, a well-honed post-run routine will help prevent injury, boost your health - and improve your running.

You can help to avoid muscle stiffness and soreness after your run by following a simple static stretching routine. Static stretching can be hard to fit in a busy schedule, but the more flexible you are, the more progress you'll make.

Do the stretches here after a training session when your muscles are still warm, as stretching when cold can risk damage. It's good to stretch on your rest days too.

100

SEATED HAMSTRING STRETCH

MUSCLES - hamstrings
EFFECT - supple hamstrings help prevent injuries in your knees, hips and lower back.
TECHNIQUE
• Sit on the floor with your left leg straight and your right leg bent.
• Reach forward with your left hand and aim to touch your toes.
• Hold the position for 30 seconds before changing over to the right.
WATCH POINTS - only reach comfortably. Over-stretching can cause injuries.

QUADRICEPS STRETCH

MUSCLES - quadriceps
EFFECT - the stronger your muscles are the tighter they will feel.
TECHNIQUE
• Lie on your left side.
• Grab hold of your right ankle with your right hand and pull your heel towards your bottom until you feel the stretch through your front thigh.
• Hold the stretch for 30 seconds before changing over to the other side.
WATCH POINTS - if you can't reach your ankle grab hold of your shoe.

CAT STRETCH

MUSCLES - back (erector spinae)
EFFECT - improve mobility in your back and reduce back pain
TECHNIQUE
• Kneel on all fours.
• Curve your spine up to form an arch.
• Hold the position for a second.
• Arch your back and make it hollow.
• Hold the position for a second.
• Alternate between the two moves.
• Repeat ten times.
WATCH POINTS - keep your arms straight.

WINDING DOWN AFTER YOUR RUN

For most runners it's all about the finishing line – training hard, racing tough and getting there as fast as you can. But instead of hurtling straight back into daily life the second your pulse has returned to normal, take time to recharge yourself physically and mentally.

BODY SCAN MEDITATION

Stress hormones such as cortisol are pumping through your body during an intense run, so calm your body afterwards with a body scan meditation. Take a few seconds to focus on each part of your body, working your way up from your feet. Focus on how each part feels; if you sense tightness or pain take in a long breath and release the tension as you breathe out.

CHILD'S POSE

MUSCLES - shoulders, back, inner thighs, top of your feet (deltoids, erector spinae, adductors, foot extensors)
EFFECT - places your spine in a natural position and is a great way to release tension. If you are very flexible you might not feel much of a stretch.
TECHNIQUE
• Sit on your knees on the floor with the top parts of your feet flat on the floor.
• Lower your head forward until it rests on the floor in front of you.
• Reach your arms as far forward as possible.
• Hold the position for 30 seconds minimum.
WATCH POINTS - stretch only as much as your body feels comfortable with.

GLUTE STRETCH

MUSCLES - glutes, hamstring
EFFECT - avoid tightness through your bottom that can lead to pain in your hips or bottom.
TECHNIQUE
• Place your left foot on your right knee.
• Keep your right leg at a right angle.
• Hold your right leg and pull your legs in towards your chest.
• You should feel a stretch in your left buttocks.
• Hold the position for 30 seconds before changing over to the right.
WATCH POINTS - keep your head relaxed on the ground.

DO THE COUNT-FIVE BREATHING EXERCISE
Release tension and regenerate your mind and body after all the exertion with some mindful breathing. Take deep in and out breaths from your belly. Count five in and five out. Take five to ten minutes to focus on your breathing.

COOL DOWN JOG
Jog lightly for a few minutes if you've done a short run, or up to a mile if you've done a longer distance or a race. This will boost recovery, flush out lactic acid and metabolic waste and bring your body back to a resting state.

DO A MINDFULNESS MEDITATION
After the race, block any thoughts of what you should or are going to do next. Instead, focus fully on the sounds you can hear, how your body feels, what you can see and smell. Engage all your senses; if you feel distracted pull yourself back to the present.

ACHILLES STRETCH

MUSCLES - achilles
EFFECT - countering the tightness through running that can lead to different injuries in the tendon.
TECHNIQUE
• Stand with your left foot slightly in front of your right. Ensure that your toes are pointing straight forward.
• Bend your knees and sit back onto your right leg.
• Push your right heel onto the ground.
• Hold the position for 30 seconds before changing over to the left.
WATCH POINTS - keep your back straight and look forward.

TAKE STOCK OF YOUR RUNNING
Once you've spent a few minutes breathing and doing your mindfulness exercises, take stock of how the run went. Don't beat yourself up; just acknowledge any feelings you have about your performance and where you want to go from here. Make a mental note of anything you can learn from the run that will help you improve next time. Give yourself a set amount of time to do this (try five minutes) rather than dwelling on it for hours, which can make you feel bad.

101

DRINK CHOCOLATE MILK
Eat something as soon as you can after intense exercise to refuel your muscles – and ideally within 40 minutes. Chocolate milk has a good ratio of protein and lactose.

HAVE YOUR SHOWER, THEN DO A LONGER MEDITATION
After you've taken your post-run shower, lie down and take 10 to 20 minutes to meditate: focus and quiet your mind – and your body. Turn off any noisy distractions, wear comfortable clothes, find a quiet place and close your eyes. Focus on your breathing. If your mind starts to wander, bring it back and attempt to clear your mind by thinking about nothing but your breathing.

TAKE A NAP
If you've the luxury of plenty of time after a run, take a nap when you get the chance. Sleep is the best recovery tool available. Elite Kenyan professional runners, who train several times a day, sleep as much and as often as they can between running sessions.

" The more flexible you are, the more progress you'll make."

FOAM ROLLER EXERCISES

Try these moves with a foam roller to release tight knots and ease tension in your muscles.

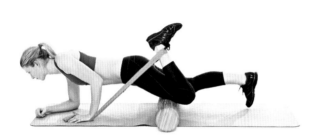

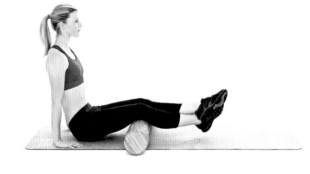

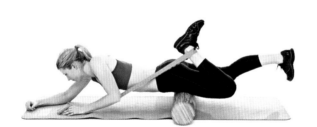

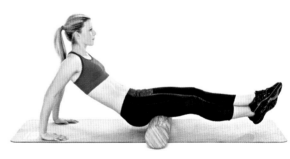

FRONT THIGH RELEASE WITH EXERCISE BAND

AREAS TRAINED - quadriceps
EFFECT - releasing tight quadriceps improves your performance.
TECHNIQUE
• Lie on your stomach and place the foam roller underneath your thighs.
• Bend your left leg and place an exercise band around your ankle.
• Pull your ankle towards your bottom with your left hand and place your hand on the floor next to your body.
• Support your body on your right forearm.
• Roll the foam roller down towards your knee.
• Roll up again, then swap sides.
WATCH POINTS - don't roll over your knee joint.

HAMSTRING RELEASE

AREAS TRAINED - hamstrings
EFFECT - helps to prevent a variety of running-related problems.
TECHNIQUE
• Sit on the floor and place the foam roller underneath your right knee.
• Place your left ankle on top of your right ankle.
• Support your upper body with your arms and lift your bottom off the floor.
• Roll yourself forwards and backwards over the foam roller.
WATCH POINTS - if you find a tender spot, hold the position for a few seconds. Be careful when rolling over the area behind the knees.

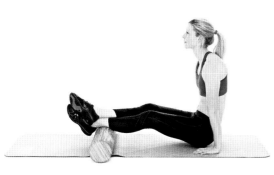

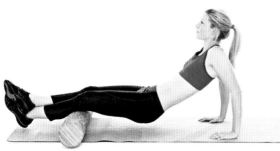

CALF RELEASE

AREAS TRAINED – gastrocnemius and soleus muscles
EFFECT – prevention of calf injuries, which will prevent you from running and can also lead to compensation injuries.
TECHNIQUE
• Sit on the floor and place the foam roller underneath your left calf.
• Place your right ankle on top of your left.
• Support your upper body with your arms and lift your bottom off the floor.
• Roll yourself forwards and backwards over the foam roller, covering the area from your knee to your ankle.
• Repeat on the right.
WATCH POINTS – if you find a tender spot in the muscle, hold the position for a few seconds. Be careful when rolling over the area behind the knees.

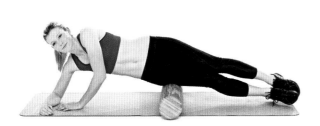

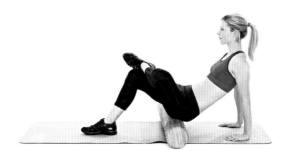

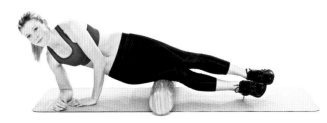

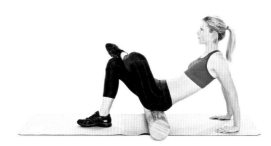

ITB RELEASE

AREAS TRAINED – iliotibial band (ITB)
EFFECT – Relieve tension that can lead to knee problems.
TECHNIQUE
• Lie with your right hip on the foam roller.
• Keep your left leg on top of your right leg.
• Support your upper body on your right forearm and your left hand.
• Use your arms to roll from your hip to your knee and back again.
• Repeat on the left side.
WATCH POINTS - don't roll over your knee joint.

GLUTE RELEASE

AREAS TRAINED – glutes
EFFECT – prevent back and knee problems, keep glutes strong and flexible.
TECHNIQUE
• Sit on the foam roller and place your hands behind you on the floor.
• Place your left foot on your right knee.
• Lean slightly over to the right.
• Roll forwards and backwards over your bottom.
• Repeat on the other side.
WATCH POINTS - keep the moves small and controlled.

30-SECOND STRETCHES

As you should know having got this far, stretching is vital. Here is a selection to do at the end of each run, holding each one for at least 30 seconds.

QUAD STRETCH

AREAS TRAINED – quadriceps
EFFECT – tightness in your front thighs can lead to knee and muscle injuries, or damage to your kneecap.
TECHNIQUE
• Standing on your right leg, grab your left ankle with your left hand.
• Pull your heel up towards your bottom, keeping your knees together.
WATCH POINTS - hold on to a secure object if you struggle to keep your balance.

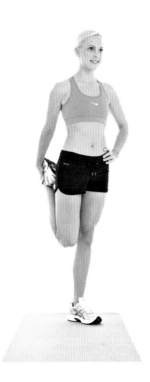

CALF STRETCH

AREAS TRAINED - Gastrocnemius muscles
EFFECT – Prevent ankle, knee and hip injuries due to tightness.
TECHNIQUE
• Place the toes of your left foot on a weight or step.
• Step forwards with your right foot and hold the stretch.
WATCH POINTS - don't bend your back knee.

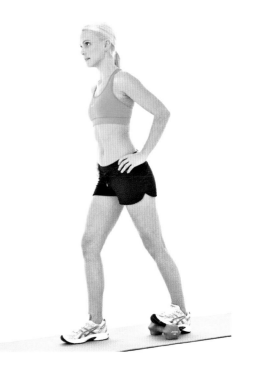

HIP FLEXOR STRETCH

AREAS TRAINED - psoas muscles
EFFECT - hip flexors lift your knees, are very small and if they get too tight can lead to pain in your hips and lower back. Hold the stretch; as it gets easier, slowly push forwards until you feel the stretch again.
TECHNIQUE
• Kneel on your left knee, placing your right foot in front of you.
• Push your hips forwards until you feel a stretch around your hips and front thigh.
• Hold the position before changing to the other side.
WATCH POINTS - pull your shoulders back and be sure not to slouch.

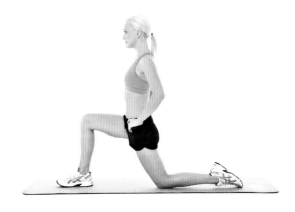

ITB STRETCH

AREAS TRAINED - Iliotibial band (ITB)
EFFECT - Stretching your ITB can reduce the pressure on your knees and help with pain on the outside of the knees.
TECHNIQUE
• Lie down on your left side.
• Place your left foot over your right knee.
• Pull your right heel up towards your bottom and push your right knee down to the floor with your left foot.
WATCH POINTS - if you're not flexible enough to get your left foot over your right knee, keep it on the floor and make sure your right knee is against the floor.

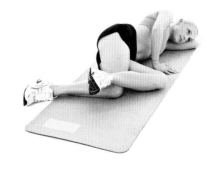

105

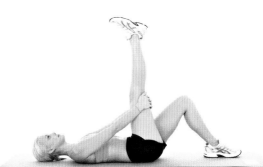

GLUTE STRETCH

AREAS TRAINED - glutes
EFFECT - your bottom works hard while you run, so it's important to have good flexibility to prevent injuries. Hold the stretch and, as it gets easier, slowly pull your leg towards you until you feel the stretch again.
TECHNIQUE
• Lie on your back.
• Place your right ankle across your left knee.
• Grabbing hold of your left thigh, pull your left knee towards your chest.
WATCH POINTS - don't "bounce" the stretch.

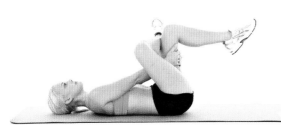

HAMSTRING STRETCH

AREAS TRAINED - hamstrings
EFFECT - keep those hamstrings flexible. Hold the stretch, and then, as it gets easier, slowly pull your leg towards you a bit more, until you feel the stretch again.
TECHNIQUE
• Lie on your back, with your left leg bent and your foot flat on the floor.
• Extend your right leg up towards the ceiling.
• Holding your right thigh, pull your leg towards your body.
WATCH POINTS - don't "bounce" the stretch.

STAY LOOSE

If you are a trail runner, these stretches should comprise a key part of your regular routine to stay loose.

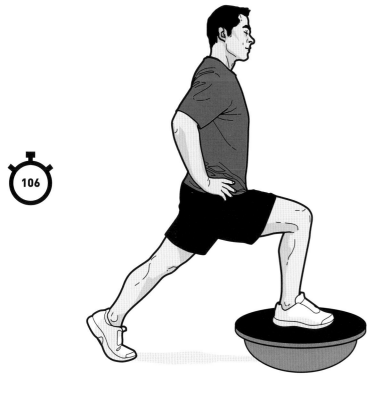

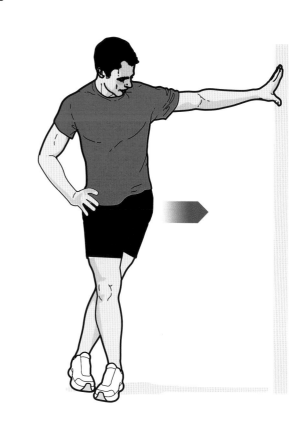

ANKLES

EFFECT - stability is more important than flexibility. Having very mobile ankles can increase injuries if you're running on uneven terrain. Stability is always more important for trail runners.

TECHNIQUE
Try some lunges on a BOSU ball, or unilateral plyometrics (a variation of hopping drills).

PIRIFORMIS

EFFECT - great release for sufferers of sciatica or piriformis syndrome. Often referred to as "the dancer's stretch".

TECHNIQUE
Keep your hips straight and your foot as parallel to your hips as you can. Hold for 60 seconds on each side and go for an 8/10 level of intensity.

WATCH POINT - do not attempt if you are experiencing any pain in your knees.

GROIN

EFFECT - actively trying to switch off your tendons' self defence mechanism.

TECHNIQUE

Self-PNF moves. Proprioceptive Neuromuscular Facilitation (PNF) is a flexibility system. Place your hands on your knees and push down while resisting with your knees. Then after ten seconds stop resisting with your knees - you will be literally forcing yourself into a more flexible state. Do this slowly at first and aim for four sets.

HIP FLEXOR

EFFECT - lengthen the top of the quads and fully stretch out the hip flexors. Tight hip flexors can really affect running biomechanics. Perform this stretch if your trail is uphill and certainly before a hill training session.

TECHNIQUE

Go into the lunge position, then grab your back foot and pull it up to your glute. Keep the body as upright as you can and slightly push out and forwards with your hips (like someone is behind you, pushing your butt forward). Do two sets of 30 seconds each side. Go for a 9/10 intensity.

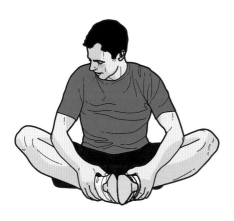

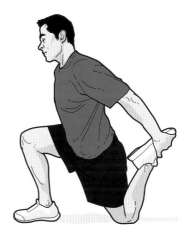

107

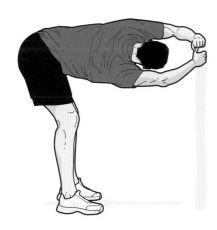

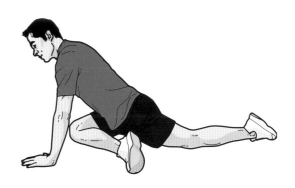

BACK

EFFECT - helps to counteract the strain of a static day job.

TECHNIQUE

Try to rotate as far as you can each side for 90 seconds, holding for ten seconds on each rotation. If you do a lot of uneven ground running, your lats and obliques will be tighter than normal.

ITB

EFFECT - getting all the knots out before a stretch.

TECHNIQUE

Use a foam roller first and then be patient. It may take you a minute to find the best angle. When you find it, push until you reach a 9/10 level of intensity. Hold for two sets of 30 seconds on each side.

STRENGTH & CONDITIONING EXERCISES

Focus on your strength and conditioning to help prevent injury to your key running muscles.

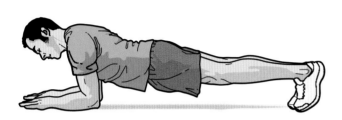

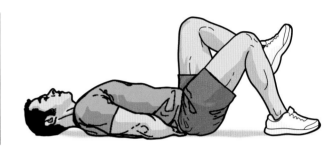

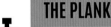

THE PLANK

TECHNIQUE
• Keep a straight line from the neck down through the legs to your ankles.
• Engage all your core muscles by sucking your belly button up to the ceiling.
• Keep your chest over your elbows.
ADVANCED VERSION – hold this for 30 seconds to one minute and build it up gradually. If this is too hard to begin with, you can avoid lower back pain by doing the move with your knees on the ground.

THE FINGER CRUSHER

TECHNIQUE
• Get into a sit-up position.
• Find the natural arch in your back.
• Place your hands under that arch.
• Engage your lower abs and pelvic floor
• Push your spine down onto your hands, trying to crush your fingers.
ADVANCED VERSION – slight alternate leg lifts, keeping the pressure on your hands even.

SPLIT-LEG LUNGE

TECHNIQUE
• To work your running muscles in a full chain movement, point your toes forward, keep your back heel lifted and with hands on hips, lunge down, squeezing the glute of your rear leg.
• Make sure everything goes down in the centre and you're not lunging forwards.
• Your knee should not be over the front of your toes.
• Lunge forward with a bent back knee.
ADVANCED VERSION – once you've nailed this move, you can progress to driving the knee up from the lunge.

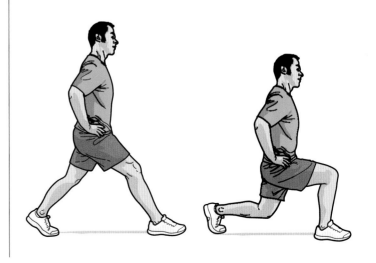

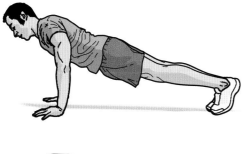

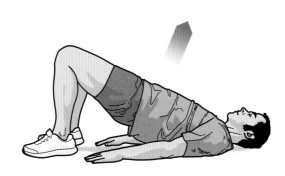

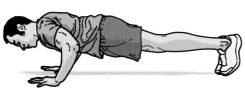

PRESS-UP

TECHNIQUE
• To improve your arm swing when running, place your hands shoulder and a half's width apart.
• Get into the plank position.
• Lower your chest to the floor and push back up, not just pushing through your chest and arms but also through your core.

THE BRIDGE

TECHNIQUE
• Get into the sit-up position
• Keep your stomach strong, engage your glutes and roll up into a bridge.
• Keep your hips high by squeezing your glute muscles.
ADVANCED VERSION – make this tougher by putting your hands over your chest.

109

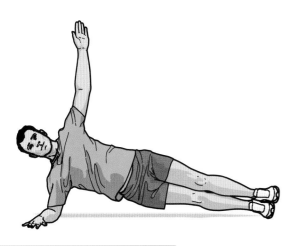

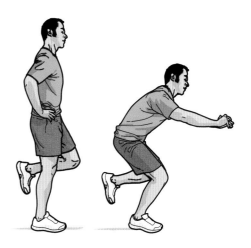

THE SIDE PLANK

TECHNIQUE
• Make a right angle with your supporting arm, your feet together and your stomach strong.
• Rise up, making sure you squeeze your glutes and pushing your pelvis through.
• Hold for 30 seconds.
ADVANCED VERSION – lift your free arm into the air, keep your side really strong, don't let your middle sag.

ONE-LEGGED SQUAT

TECHNIQUE
• Another way of working your muscles in a full chain movement; stand on one leg, engaging your glute on your standing leg and keep your hips facing forward and aligned with your knee and toe.
• Go down as far as you can without allowing your knee to roll inwards.
ADVANCED VERSION – use a stability ball between yourself and a wall for balance in the early stages.

PLYOMETRIC EXERCISES

This mix of strengthening and plyometric moves is useful for those who are heading out to run on trails.

Plyometric exercises are designed to improve your explosive power – ideal when you're looking to add some speed and strength to your running. Coupled with some top strengthening moves, plyometrics are also the perfect exercises to do before trail running, as they will get your fast-twitch muscles into gear, making your legs feel more responsive. Trail running places greater demands on your body than road running, so it helps if you're agile, in order to be able to change direction quickly to avoid rocks and stones, duck down to avoid branches, and leap from side to side to prevent tripping over tree roots or incur wet feet stepping in puddles.

With all these hazards potentially occurring within a short distance, it helps if you are flexible enough to prevent injury caused by any sudden movements you may need to make. To run trails effectively and remain injury free, you need a workout routine that hones your reaction times, boosts your coordination and balance, and improves your flexibility.

GLUTE STEP-UP CIRCUIT

TECHNIQUE
• Stand on a step or bench on your left leg, with your right leg hanging off the side of the step.
• Squeeze the glutes of your standing leg, to control the movement, and hitch your free hip up, so your hips are at an angle.
• Swing your free leg out to the side as high as you can, before lowering it back down with control.
• Maintaining the angle in your hips (keeping your free hip hitched up), immediately perform a squat on the standing leg, ensuring your knee doesn't go over your toes.
• Repeat ten to 20 times standing on your left leg, before switching over to your right.

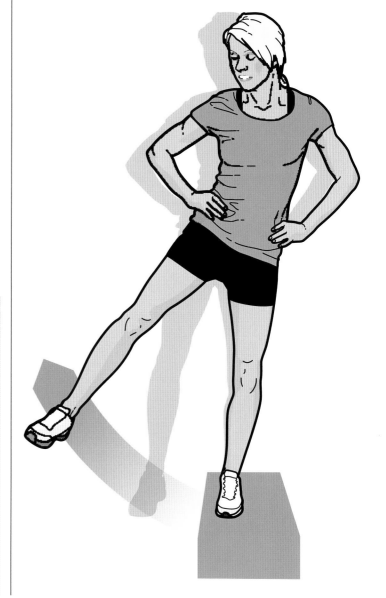

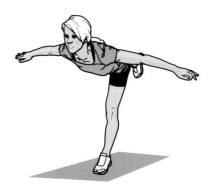

HAMSTRING STEP AND BOW

TECHNIQUE
• Step forward with your left leg, then, as you pivot from your hip, lean forward so your upper body is parallel with the ground and your right leg is raised behind you.
• Squeeze your glutes and hamstrings and bring your body back to an upright position, then immediately step forward with your right leg and repeat the move, this time raising your left leg out behind you.
• Repeat the move for 20 to 30 steps.

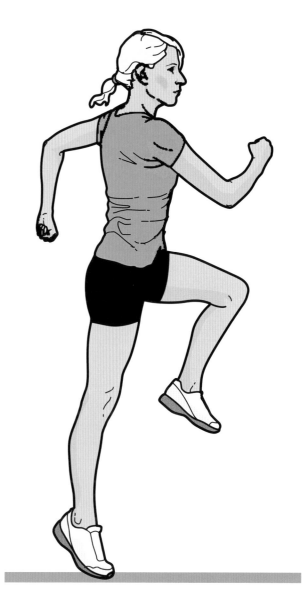

111

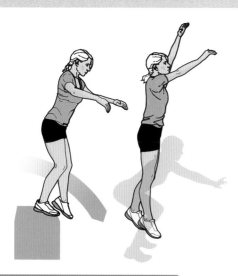

DEPTH JUMPS

TECHNIQUE
• Stand on a step or bench.
• Step off the bench with one leg, with your feet active (flexed).
• Your feet should meet in the air, then land on both feet.
• As soon as you land, rebound back off the floor into a jump.
• Make sure you have as short a contact time with the floor as possible and bounce as high as you can.
• Repeat five to ten times.

HIGH-KNEE WALK WITH GLUTE HOLD

TECHNIQUE
• As you walk forward in this slow and exaggerated walk, lift your knees up high.
• Focus on squeezing your glutes as you lift each knee in turn and hold the top position for a second or two while your knee is in the air.
• Keep your shoulders relaxed.
• Suck your tummy in to promote a strong core.
• Walk forward for 20 to 30 steps.

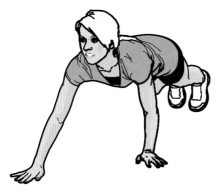

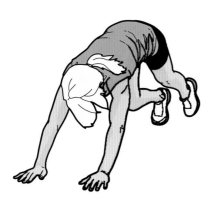

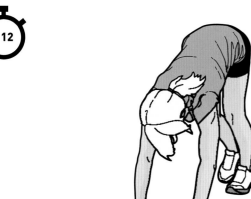

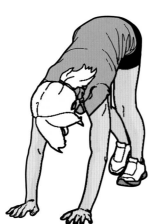

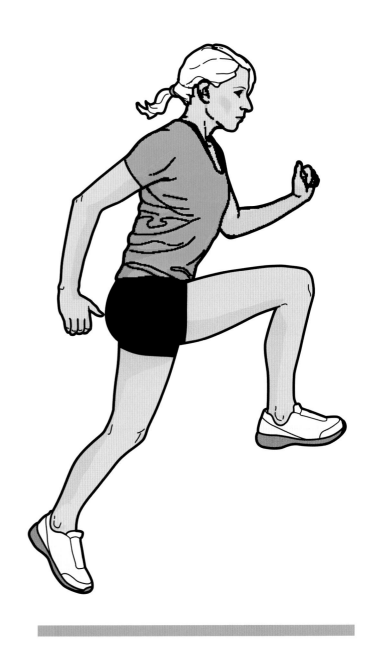

JUMPING SPLIT SQUATS

AREAS TRAINED - glutes and hip flexors
Effect -power exercise, particularly good for hills.
TECHNIQUE
• Starting in a lunge position, with left foot forward and right foot back, jump up very powerfully, high and quick.
• Land with feet in the opposite positions - right foot forward and left foot back.
• Do this continually for 60 seconds.
• Repeat for two sets.

HIGH-KNEE RUNNING

TECHNIQUE
• Run forwards with an exaggerated high-knee running action, making sure you maintain an upright posture and put a spring in your step.
• Ensure you lift your knees up high, keeping your feet active and pump your arms forwards and backwards.
• Run forwards for 30 steps.

BLIND LINEAR HOPS

TECHNIQUE
• Get a marker that's low off the ground, such as a rolled-up towel and hop with one leg back and forth over it.
• As soon as you get into the rhythm, close your eyes; see if you can get to 20 without falling over, opening your eyes or landing on the towel.

WATCH POINT
Any activity with your eyes shut adds an extra element of danger, so ensure you have plenty of space. With your eyes closed your body will be forced to use its natural awareness to stay balanced and coordinated. The better balance you have, the less likely you are to trip on your runs. In addition, all hopping will increase ankle-tendon and calf-muscle strength

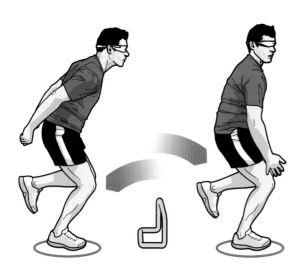

CATERPILLAR WALK

TECHNIQUE
• To work your whole body, with emphasis on your core, place your hands and feet on the floor.
• Walk your hands out, so that you are in a plank position.
• Walk your feet towards your hands.
• As your toes touch the floor, push your heel to the ground, so you feel the stretch in your hamstrings.
• Once your feet are right behind your hands and your legs are straight, walk your hands forward into a plank.
• Repeat this move five to ten times.

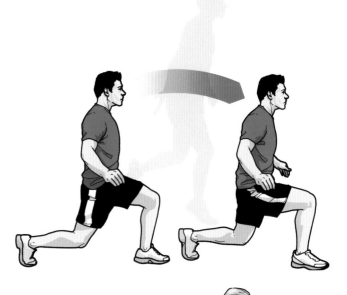

113

LATERAL SINGLE-LEG HOPS

TECHNIQUE
• With one foot always off the floor, jump from side to side over a line.
• Do the hops as quickly as you can, two sets of 40 for each leg. This will improve foot speed, calf power and coordination, ideal for those sharp turns and tree-root evasions.

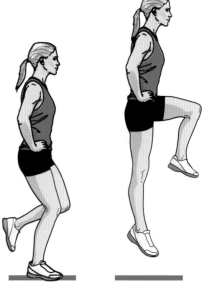

The exercises in this part of the programme will enhance your brain's ability to control your muscles quickly, which will help keep you on your feet, while also encouraging improvements in coordination, flexibility and quick response times.

You can begin on flat ground and then progress to trying the hops on an uneven surface, for even greater benefits to your strength and proprioception – the link between your mind and body.

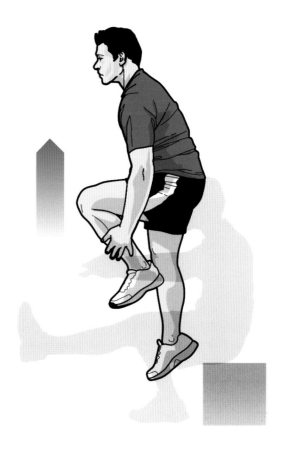

BENCH "PLYO" PISTOL SQUATS

AREA TRAINED – leg strength
EFFECT – power-building to a greater extent than basic squats, fully activating the glutes, which can be the cause of many injuries.
TECHNIQUE
• Begin in a one-legged squat, with a bench behind you.
• As soon as your bottom touches the bench, drive up straight, using your base leg, with sufficient force that you hop up, rather than just standing up quickly.
• Land and repeat the move.
• Do six sets of 20. Change feet after each set.

114

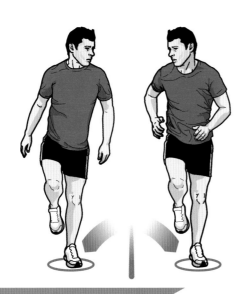

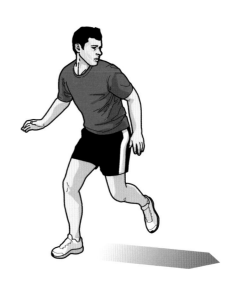

SIDE-STEPPING

AREAS TRAINED – core, abductors and obliques and training knees in lateral movement.
EFFECT – injury prevention.
TECHNIQUE
• Keep your feet facing the same way as your hips.
• Sidestep for four sets of 100 metres.
• Switch the lead leg after each set.
• Start slowly and build up speed.

TWO-FOOTED JUMP TO SINGLE-LEG LANDING

TECHNIQUE
• Stand with your feet hip-width apart.
• Jump sideways as far as you can but land on just one foot, with power and balance; your ankle and knee stabiliser muscles will be working hard.
• Do four sets of 20 reps. Change feet after each set.

BOUNCY BALL TENNIS

TECHNIQUE
• Find a wall with some open space in front of it.
• Throw a tennis ball against the wall, then run to where it returns so you can hit it back to the wall.
• Repeat for as long as you can continue the "rally" and aim to move the ball around, so you have to run, twist, reach or jump to hit the next shot.

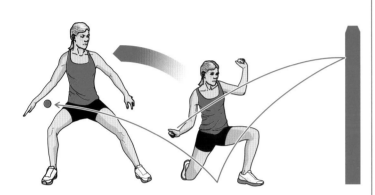

CRISS-CROSS HOPS

TECHNIQUE
• Stand on your right leg – the point where you're standing is your start and finish point and is the centre of an imaginary cross.
• First hop forwards, then hop back to the start point, then hop to the right, returning to the start point, to the back, returning to the start point, and to the left, returning to the start point.
• Switch to your left leg and repeat the process.
• Rest and then repeat on each leg five times.

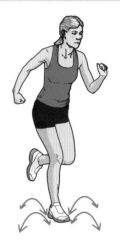

115

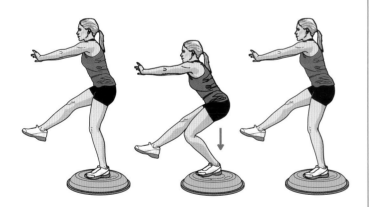

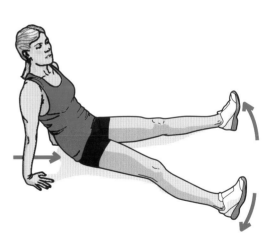

SINGLE-LEG SQUATS ON WOBBLE BOARD

TECHNIQUE
• Stand on your right leg, while holding your left leg out a little in front of you.
• Sit into a single-leg squat.
• Move slowly and hold your position at the bottom of the squat for two seconds.
• Repeat for five squats on this leg before swapping to the left leg and performing the same action.

THIGH STRETCH

TECHNIQUE
• Sit on the floor with your legs out wide in front of you.
• Use your arms to slide your bottom forwards and let your feet drift a little further apart.
• As your feet move apart, you'll feel an increased stretch along the length of your inner thighs.
• Hold this position for ten seconds, relax and repeat three times.

CORE STRENGTH EXERCISES

You can help your core muscles to support your running by using exercises targeted at that key part of the runner's anatomy.

Your stomach and back form the centre point of your running. Without a strong core, your arm and leg movements can't work together as an effective unit. Do three sets of 15 to 20 repetitions of any of these ideas.

Perform any three exercises each day, and ensure you complete all of the exercises at least once a week. You'll need 2.5 kg dumbbells, a stability ball, exercises bands and a mat.

BENCH PRONE ROW

AREA TRAINED - rhomboids
EFFECT - trained upper back improves both posture and lung capacity.
TECHNIQUE
• Lie on your stomach on a bench, holding a weight in each hand, palms facing your feet.
• Pull your hands up towards your armpits.
• Lower your hands back down to the floor.
WATCH POINTS - squeeze your shoulder blades together in the raised position.

STABILITY BALL BACK EXTENSION

AREA TRAINED - erector spinae
EFFECT - the stability ball not only increases core strength but improves balance and coordination.
TECHNIQUE
• Lie on your stomach on a stability ball, crossing your arms in front of you.
• Lift your head and shoulders about three to four inches off the ball (if you feel yourself rolling backwards, make this movement smaller).
• Slowly return to the starting position.
WATCH POINTS - keep your knees slightly bent to help you keep your balance, make sure your movements are small and controlled.

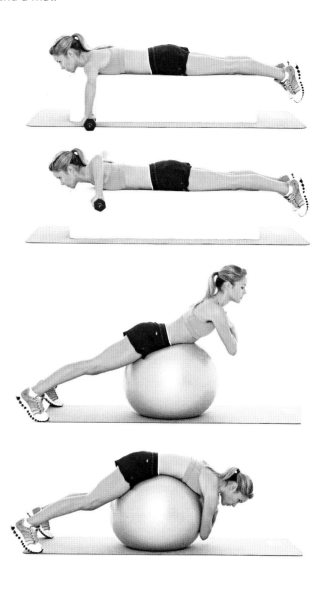

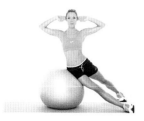
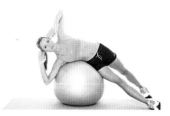
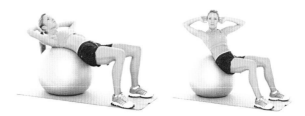

STABILITY BALL SIDE-LIFT

AREA TRAINED – obliques
EFFECT – making more efficient rotation in your hips and shoulders.
TECHNIQUE
• With your feet securely against a wall for balance, place your hip on the stability ball, with your bottom leg forwards and your top leg backwards.
• Lower yourself over the ball, then lift up as high as you can.
• Hold the top position for a second before lowering your body once more over the ball.
WATCH POINTS – keep your feet wide apart to aid your balance; the closer the ball is to the wall, the harder the exercise.

STABILITY BALL CROSS-OVER

AREA TRAINED – transversus abdominis, rectus abdominis and obliques
EFFECT – stomach strength, balance and coordination.
TECHNIQUE
• Lie with your lower back supported on the ball and place your hands on your temples.
• Crunch your head and shoulders up while twisting over to your right side.
• Lower back down to the starting position.
• Repeat the move towards your left side.
WATCH POINTS – don't lift more than two to three inches.

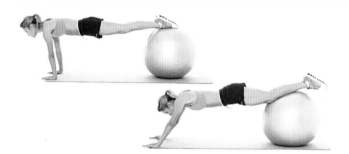

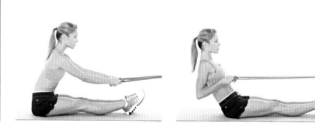

117

STABILITY BALL PUSH-BACK

AREA TRAINED – erector spinae, rectus abdominis and transversus abdominis
EFFECT – functional exercise to help you use back and stomach muscles as a unit.
TECHNIQUE
• Place your hands on the floor, with your feet on a stability ball.
• Push your body backwards, allowing the ball to roll back (keep your belly pulled in towards your spine to stop your back arching as you roll).
• Making sure you keep your hands in the same position throughout the movement, roll forwards back to the starting position.
WATCH POINTS – be safe: if you feel any pain in your lower back, lift your glutes higher to stop your back arching.

SEATED ELASTIC-BAND ROW

AREA TRAINED – erector spinae
EFFECT – your stronger back means you won't lean forwards when you run.
TECHNIQUE
• Tie an exercise band close to the ground around a secure object.
• Sitting on the floor with your legs straight, hold the ends of the band so that you can feel the tension.
• Lean forwards from your waist, maintaining the resistance in the exercise band.
• Lean backwards, to about 110 degrees, pulling your hands in towards your chest and squeezing your shoulder blades.
• Hold for a second before repeating.
WATCH POINTS – use an exercise band that provides sufficient resistance or use the pulley machine in the gym.

AVOID AND BEAT ILLNESS

Know when to run, when to take time out and how to prevent the need to take a running sickie.

Whether you're following a training schedule for a race or are just motivated to run regularly, it can be very frustrating to get ill. You don't want to miss your run but neither do you want to make things worse and risk putting yourself out of action for longer. The right thing to do is not always obvious, but you can look for the signs.

SIMPLE COLD
OK TO RUN – your nose is a bit runny or stuffed up and you have a mild headache or a slight sore throat. All your symptoms are above your neck.
MISS YOUR RUN – your nose is streaming, you have a high temperature, you feel shivery, your joints or muscles ache and you need regular paracetamol.

COUGH
OK TO RUN – your cough is dry and tickly and the irritation is in your throat. You don't have a temperature and are only coughing occasionally.
MISS YOUR RUN – your cough feels like it's coming from your chest and is producing phlegm. You feel short of breath or wheezy. You have a temperature.

SORE THROAT
OK TO RUN – your throat feels dry and a bit scratchy, but it isn't too painful to swallow and you otherwise feel fine.
MISS YOUR RUN – you have a temperature or feel shivery. Your glands are swollen, making your neck feel stiff. It hurts a lot to swallow.

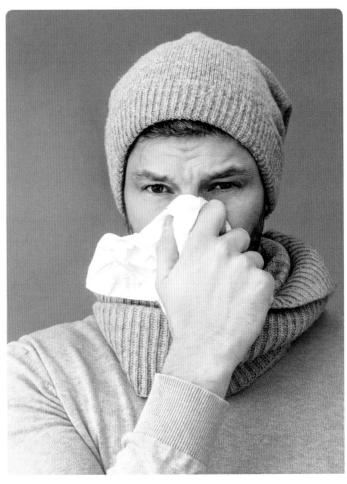

INFECTION
OK TO RUN – your sinuses feel mildly congested and a bit tender but you feel fine otherwise and you can breathe easily.
MISS YOUR RUN – you feel lightheaded or dizzy. You have a temperature or feel shivery. Your face or teeth are hurting.

DIARRHOEA
OK TO RUN – you have just had one or two small bouts of loose stools and you don't feel that there'll be more. You don't feel sick or have tummy pain, you've drunk plenty of fluids and have had something to eat.
MISS YOUR RUN – you're getting stomach cramps and know there is more diarrhoea to come. You feel sick or have vomited, have a temperature, haven't eaten and you're a bit dehydrated.

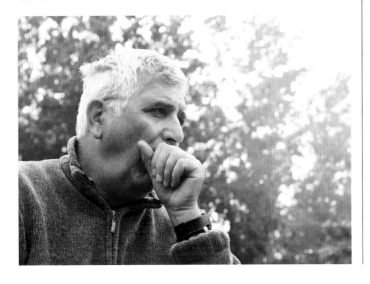

URINARY INFECTION

OK TO RUN – it's a bit uncomfortable when you pass urine and you are doing so a bit more often than usual, but you feel well and don't have a tummy ache or a temperature.
MISS YOUR RUN – you feel shivery, have a stomach ache, lower-back pain or feel sick. It stings when you pass urine or it contains blood.

FLU

OK TO RUN – never.
MISS YOUR RUN – with full-blown flu you'll struggle to get out of bed, let alone run and you shouldn't even consider exercising. Don't attempt a run until you feel fully recovered and can cope easily with your normal daily life.

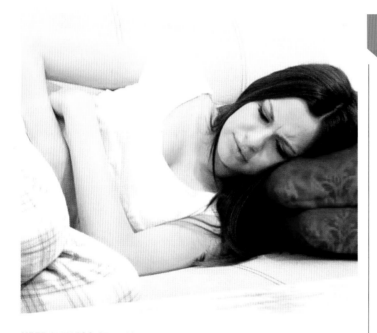

KEEP ILLNESS AT BAY

You can help your body fight off the bugs by making clever food choices. Nutritionist Kate Butler said, "Foods packed with immune-system supporting vitamins A and C are important as they're rich in antioxidants, beta carotene and vitamin E." These might include butternut squash, lemons, protein, chilli and manuka honey. Whole natural foods are good, including vegetables (particularly brightly-coloured varieties), beans, wholegrains, fruits, seeds and nuts. Even relatively small amounts of sugar can reduce the level of white blood cells needed to fight bacteria.

" You don't want to miss your run but neither do you want to make things worse."

TAKE YOUR TIME OUT SERIOUSLY

If you do have to miss a run, it's important that you rest and take it easy. Your immune system is working hard to fight the infection that has struck you down. Putting extra strain on your body by running can reduce your immune response and make you worse, as well as hampering your recovery.

When you think you're OK to run, go out with cautious attitude. Start slowly and take it easy. Stay hydrated. Don't aim for a PB, hill session or threshold run. If you do feel OK you can step things up a little, but be sensible.

HANGOVER RUNNING

Sometimes poor health may be self-inflicted... There are a few simple measures you can take to avoid your evening out becoming a blur. "You'll slow down intoxication if you have a full stomach, rather than drinking when hungry, which will allow quicker absorption," said nutritionist Daisy Connor. "The best foods and drinks to focus on are those that promote liver function and protection from free-radical damage – plenty of fresh vegetables and leafy greens, with protein (eggs, meat, fish, beans and lentils). Avoid refined carbohydrates, favouring wholefoods, since many types of alcohol are high in carbohydrate or sugar." Alternate alcoholic drinks with water or soft drinks to help reduce alcohol consumption and stave off dehydration.

"If you drank in a sensible way (a couple of drinks with food), then running should be beneficial, raising your metabolic rate and increasing oxygen intake to help with detoxification," Daisy said. "Bear in mind that anything over six units (two large glasses of wine or three double spirits) in a session is classed as binge drinking. Running with a hangover does have the potential to be damaging. Exhaustive exercise generates free radicals, as does excessive alcohol consumption. Regularly doing both could leave the body vulnerable to disease in the long term, because if you don't have enough antioxidants to counteract free radical production, cells can be damaged."

Make sure you fuel up and hydrate in the hours before the run with a protein- and nutrient-rich breakfast. Have plenty of wholegrain carbohydrates to keep your energy levels up.

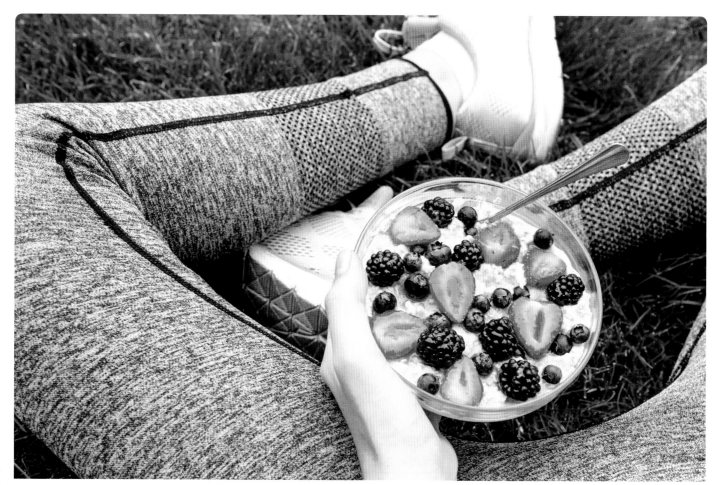

Naturopath Lina Swailem recommended potent antimicrobial foods to help fight infections. "Garlic, onions, horseradish, oregano, thyme, lemon, lime, ginger, cinnamon and cayenne pepper." Health and fitness expert Tom Eastham said that runners need their seven or nine a day rather than five. "Blueberries, kale, prunes, matcha powder, pinto beans and artichokes have high levels of antioxidants to boost your immune system. Omega 3 is possibly the best all-round supplement to take [1,000 mg of EPA Omega 3 a day] and Vitamin D3 is vital for performance and recovery." Echinacea is another way of helping to fight off colds and flu. "Runners can be more vulnerable to bugs when training for an event or if they're beginners, as the extra effort can lessen their immune function," said Ali Cullen, a nutritional therapist.

THINK POSITIVELY

"Being exposed to viruses doesn't mean you'll get ill – if your immune system is robust, it may withstand infection and speed recovery," said Dr Nerina Ramlakhan, a sleep and energy therapist. "Eat carefully, exercise regularly, sleep well and practise deep abdominal breathing to boost your parasympathetic nervous system, responsible for immunity. And think happy thoughts – optimistic people have stronger immune systems!"

Tom Eastham said that runners must recognise the toll that training takes. "Running is one of the most exhausting movements the human body can do and this depletes various essential nutrients and fluids, such as water, salt and glycogen. Your recovery should comprise good nutrition and good sleep." Dr Juliet McGrattan has also stressed the importance of sleep. "Being over-tired lowers the body's immune defence, leaving you open to infection." Adults are recommended to get around eight hours sleep per night, so one straightforward tip is to try to get to bed early.

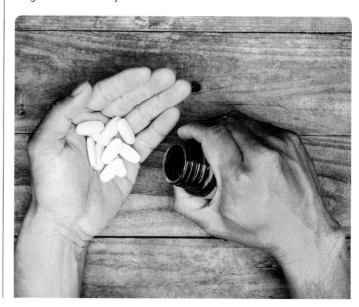

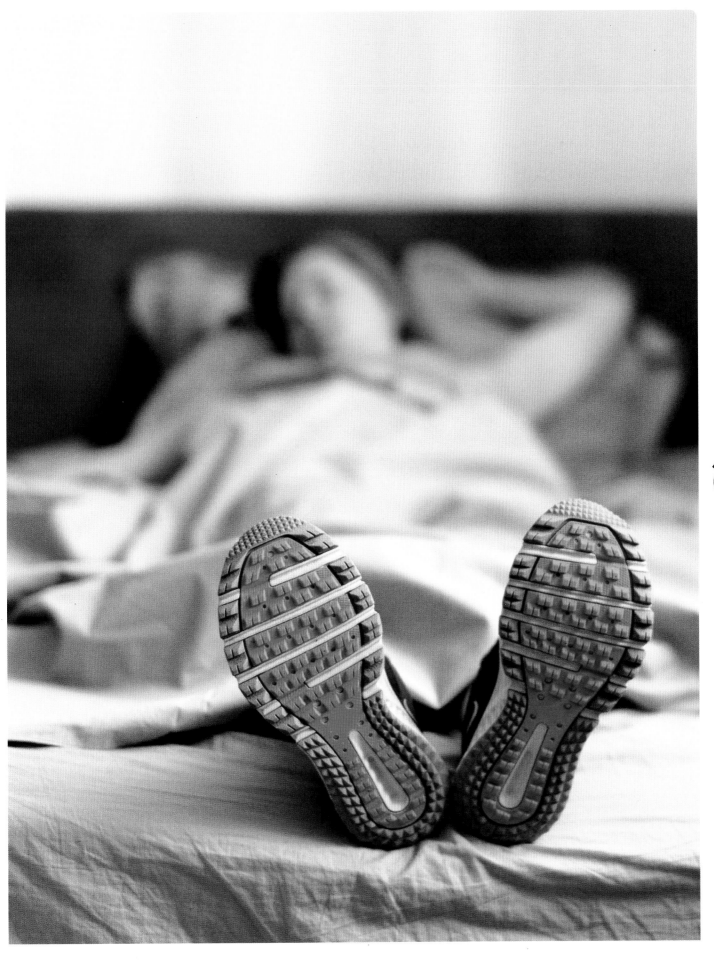

RECOVERY TIPS

As training loads go up, your legs need more than a post-run rest. Massages and cooling down gradually can both help.

If you're in the middle of a training schedule that has you out on the road three or more times a week your legs will be taking a great deal of strain. You should be doing mobilising exercises before every run and stretching properly afterwards, but sometimes something extra such a sports massage can help to keep you supple and help you recover.

Physiotherapist Paul Hobrough said, "Think of your muscle fibres as strands of hair. At one end of the scale you've got the shampoo-advert model; every strand is separate and looks beautiful in its own right. Then, at the other end, you've got something that looks like Bob Marley's dreadlocks: thick and matted. Somewhere in between will be most runners' muscles ... massaging, stretching, foam-rolling, core-conditioning and recovery runs take you closer to the shampoo model. Massage makes muscle able to build strength in the right way. In the calf you've got the gastrocnemius and soleus behind it. They do sometimes work together but they also have independent roles and if they are allowed to bond to each other it means they will both always be working."

FIBRE POWER

Muscle fibres work like a light switch – they're either on or off. When you run, it's like a relay race between muscle fibres. "In order to propel you forward, the requisite number of fibres will fire at 100 per cent, then they rest while the next part fires,' explained Hobrough. "Your fitness is measured by the speed at which that muscle fibre can recover before it's needed again."

But if a muscle is forced to fire again and again before it has had a chance to recover, fatigue will eventually set in, and that's where breakdown starts to occur. Hobrough said: "Massage helps repair those fibres in the right way to keep them in the right alignment and stop them gluing themselves to their neighbours for support. Then you can use them again the next day or the day after. Sports massage should be a little bit painful. If it's not, you're just having a relaxing massage, it's not getting into the depth you need. You've just battered your muscles so it shouldn't be over-painful. It should be more about flushing out those waste products, helping recovery. If you then stood in an ice bucket you would probably be able to run the next morning feeling very good."

MASSAGE AND YOU

Hobrough works from a simple equation that he says works for the elite athletes he treats as well as it does for hobby runners: divide the number of training sessions per week (excluding recovery and core sessions) by two. For example, three runs per week divided by two would be one and a half. You'd round down to one massage a month. Do your homework, consulting industry bodies to find a good practitioner. You want to find specialists in running injuries. Ask your local running club or specialist running shop for a recommendation. A physiotherapist who offers sports massages might be a good choice.

JUST COOL IT

Cooling down by gradually reducing the pace of your run can help prevent injury and reduce recovery time between runs. It is possible to minimise post-run leg muscle ache and in many cases eradicate it altogether. All you need to do is make sure you spend some time cooling down following every workout. Cooling down helps your heart rate and breathing return to normal gradually and can help remove waste products, such as lactic acid, which can build up during vigorous exercise.

Running causes micro trauma to muscle fibres and if you're exercising to a reasonable intensity you'll experience a build-up of lactic acid in muscles. Both are physiologically normal processes – muscle fibres are overloaded and damaged when we exercise, which is

"Massage helps repair those fibres in the right way to keep them in the right alignment and stop them gluing themselves to their neighbours for support."

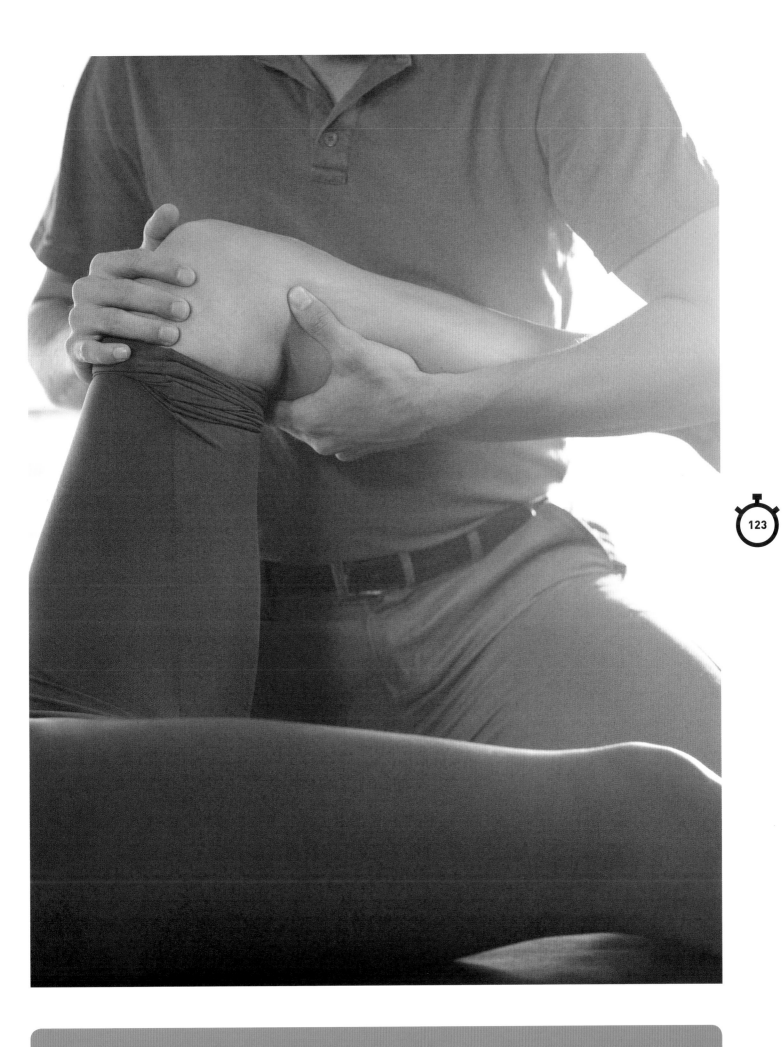

123

124

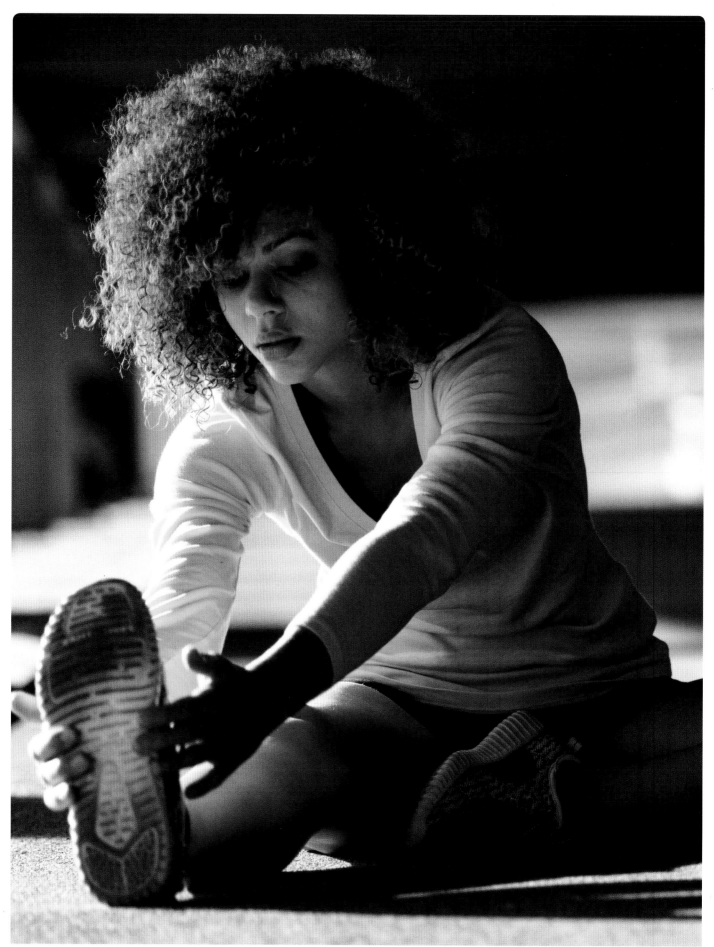

what encourages them to grow back stronger between workouts, and lactic acid is created when we increase exercise intensity sufficiently to create an environment where our muscles are working without oxygen. The two processes are essential parts of how we develop our fitness and endurance. Problems can arise, however, when we challenge the body like this but don't give it a chance to recover. The aches can then continue until the next workout, so that over time your performance and progress can be impeded or, worse, you run the risk of getting injured.

Your recovery time is every bit as important as the time you spend running, so always decrease the intensity of your run gradually. Never stop running suddenly and head straight for the shower as an abrupt end to your run can cause blood pooling in the legs, resulting in dizziness or fainting. Over a period of four to eight minutes, slow down to a jog, then a brisk walk and then, ultimately, a slow walk. This gives the muscles that have been contracting vigorously a chance to lengthen out a little and begin the recovery process before they return to pre-exercise activity levels.

DO SOMETHING DIFFERENT
Incorporate an activity other than running as part of your cool down. This minimises the damage that can be caused by exercising using muscles for one single activity. Try introducing a few minutes of cycling, cross training, rowing or swimming at the end of each run, to keep the blood circulating around the body and thoroughly clear any lingering lactic acid and other toxins from your muscles.

As we've said throughout this book, stretch after every workout. As you run, muscle fibres contract and tighten. If you don't encourage them to lengthen again following your run, they'll remain tight and this will cause you discomfort for a day or two as you go about your regular daily movements. Always leave at least five minutes at the end of each run to stretch out all the major muscle groups. Refuel promptly following each run. Eating soon after a run provides your body with the nourishment to repair muscles and recover properly. All bodily functions also require water and that includes repairing damaged muscle tissue. Drink 250–500 ml of water in the 60 to 90 minutes following your run, to ensure effective recovery.

" Decrease the intensity of your run gradually. Stopping abruptly can make you dizzy. "

125

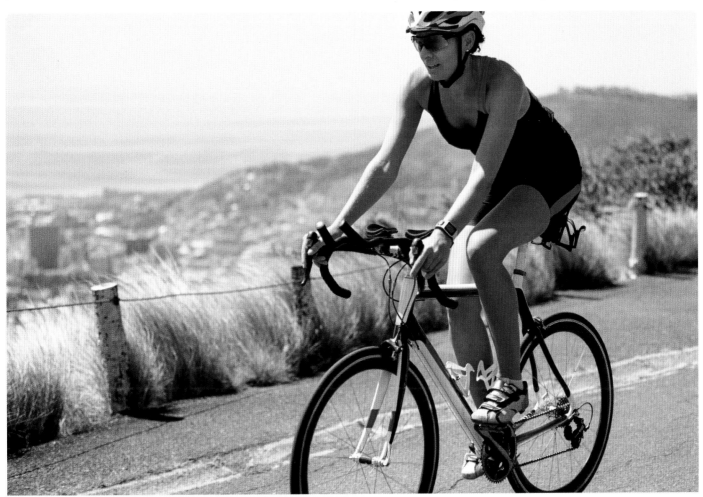

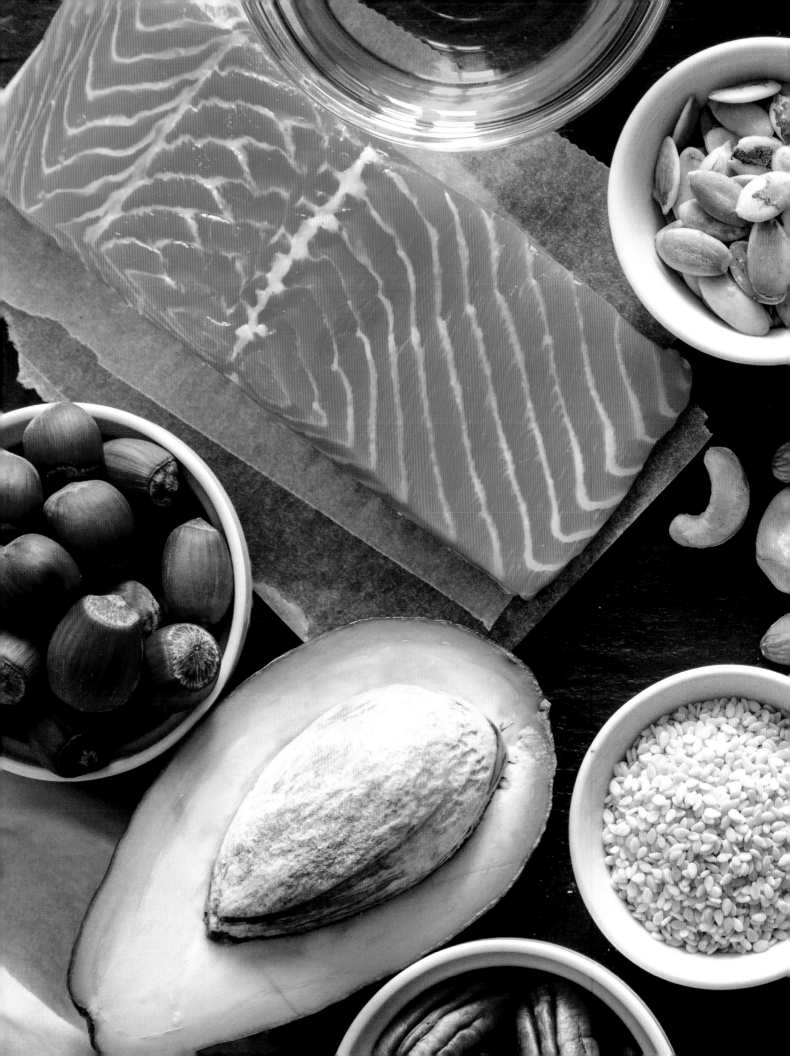

FOOD & NUTRITION

Fuel your body correctly, take on the right amount of hydration and you'll go far. You need to pay close attention to what goes into your body to make it work efficiently and to be sure that you get to the weight you want to and maintain it.

THE IMPORTANCE OF NUTRITION

A good diet is just as important as good training. Make sure you get the basics right.

Whether you decide to run for weight loss, competition, fun or fitness, you need to fuel your body correctly. Get your nutrition right and you will perform better, recover faster and stay injury-free. Even if you are running primarily to lose weight you still need to take in sufficient calories to fuel your body.

Body composition measuring devices at gyms can be used to indicate your basal metabolic rate (how many calories you need to simply fuel your body if you're doing nothing all day except existing). You then need to add on an activity factor to calculate your everyday calorie needs. This can range from 1.2 to 1.7 depending on how active you are – a nutritionist or personal trainer should be able to guide you.

To this figure you add the calories for your running or training sessions (approximately a hundred calories per mile or 4–600 calories per hour). Heart rate monitors can tell you exactly how many calories you've burned during a run or exercise session, while gym machines such as treadmills and steppers are also reasonably accurate. But if this seems too complicated, the simplest way to know if your calorie intake matches your expenditure is to monitor your weight. If you're looking to lose weight, aim to keep weight loss to something just under a kilogram per week. Otherwise, a stable weight means you're doing well.

CARBOHYDRATE NEEDS

Carbohydrates are a vital energy source for runners. Glucose derived from carbohydrates is the main type of sugar in the blood and is the body's preferred source of energy. However, we can only store relatively small amounts of glucose in our muscles and liver as glycogen.

128

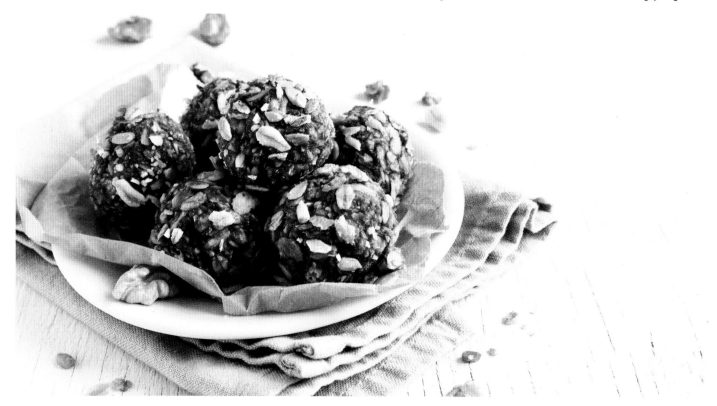

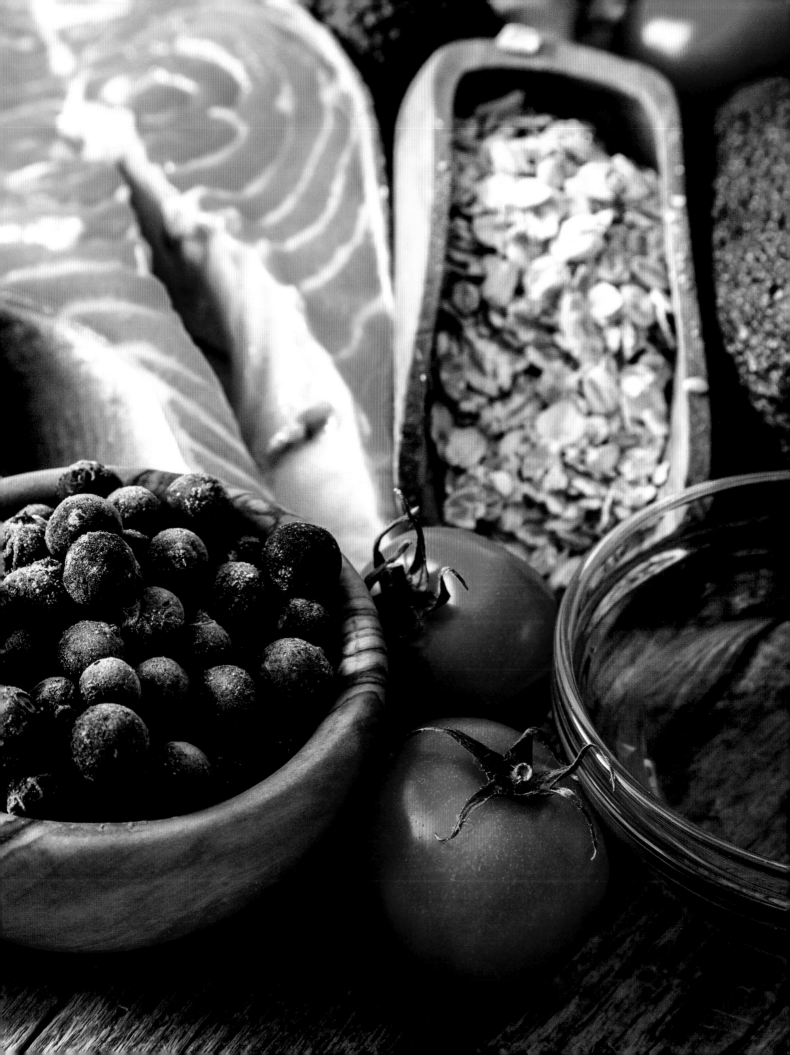

The more glycogen available, the longer you can keep going at a higher level of performance. Hitting the wall occurs as your carbohydrate reserves run low and your muscles start to use fat as an additional source of energy.

As you train more and increase your running distance, your muscles become better at transforming carbs and fat into energy, which means you can run faster for longer. The amount of carbohydrate-containing foods you eat can influence the amount of glycogen you store. Taking in sufficient carbohydrate before, during and after exercise provides glucose for energy and helps to speed up recovery and restore glycogen levels so that you're ready for your next training session.

CARBOHYDRATE SOURCES

To keep your energy levels high and avoid energy dips, eat foods that are good sources of carbohydrates, such as wholegrains – from bread, rice, cereal and pasta – as well as fruits and vegetables and some low-fat dairy foods. Most of the time focus on foods with a low glycaemic index – these foods are broken down by the body into glucose at a slower rate, providing more sustained energy. Good examples include porridge oats, wholegrain rice, rye bread, oatcakes, sweet potato and starchy vegetables.

Just before and after training you may need a more rapid energy boost to fuel your training as well as speed up recovery. This is the time to eat quick-releasing, carbohydrate-rich foods such as bananas, cereal bars, dried fruit or fruit smoothies.

GET THE RIGHT FATS

As you increase your running distance, fats become particularly important in your diet as an additional fuel. Medium chain triglycerides, found in coconut oil, for example, can be useful, as they are preferentially burnt by the body and used for energy production. As you increase your mileage try adding a spoonful of coconut oil to your morning smoothie.

All runners need to get the essential omega 3 and omega 6 fatty acids from their diet because they cannot be made in the body. Omega 3 fats, in particular, are often low in people's diets yet are hugely important for runners. These fats support tissue growth and repair, promote the production of anti-inflammatory chemicals and reduce the risk of cell damage. They may also aid recovery. To get enough essential fats, try to eat:

• two or three portions of oily fish (salmon, trout, herring, anchovy, mackerel, sardines) per week. Canned tuna is not a good source of omega 3 fats and fresh tuna can be contaminated by dioxins and mercury so limit consumption. (For more information on fish oils and how they can benefit your running, turn to page 88).
• one to two tablespoons of mixed seeds (sesame, pumpkin, sunflower, chia, flaxseed) daily. Eat these as a snack or add them to porridge, smoothies, muesli etc.
• monounsaturated fats, found in olive oil, nuts, seeds and avocados, which also possess anti-inflammatory properties.
• use olive oil and coconut oil daily in cooking, dressings or add to dishes.
• snack on nuts rich in monounsaturated fats.
• include avocado, olives, nut and seed butters regularly.

DON'T SKIMP ON YOUR PROTEIN

Pretty much everything in the body is made of proteins, which are also essential for repair. Running – especially long-distance running – can cause damage to the muscles, joints and other tissues, so ensuring sufficient protein in your diet becomes a priority.

Guidelines for daily protein intake for runners will vary depending on the amount of training you're doing. An easy way to manage your protein intake is to aim for 15–20 grams of protein at each meal and to include some protein foods with your snacks too. Good sources include lean

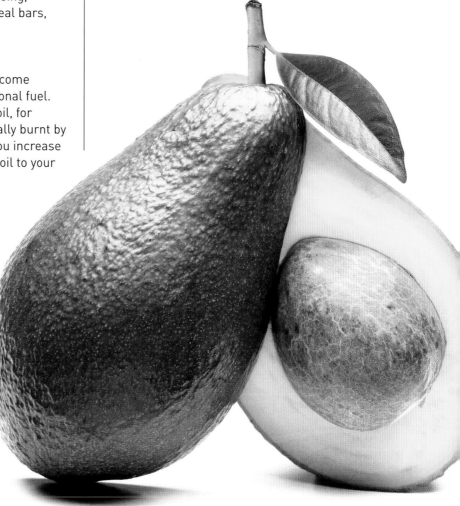

GET THE TIMING RIGHT

It's not just what you eat that makes a difference to your performance but when you eat.

BEFORE – for runs of less than an hour, focus on eating some high-carbohydrate foods about 30 minutes before training – this could mean a small, easily digested carbohydrate snack such as a banana, cereal bar or sports drink. For longer runs, eat a larger carbohydrate-based meal about two hours before training to avoid feeling nauseous during the session. This may be a bowl of porridge with some fruit and a handful of nuts and seeds.

During – if you are running for longer than one hour you may need to keep your blood glucose and fluid levels topped up. On average, runners use 60 grams of carbohydrate per hour so, depending on the length of your run, you may wish to take an isotonic drink or sports gel with you.

AFTER – to avoid energy dips and fatigue you need to replace glycogen stores, which requires carbohydrates, but you also need to promote muscle and tissue repair, which requires protein. Without correct refuelling you are less likely to get the most from your training. You may also find your next run feels harder and over time your performance may suffer. You are also more likely to develop muscle soreness and injury. Aim to eat a high-carbohydrate snack with some protein within 30–45 minutes after your run. Good examples include a protein fruit-smoothie, cereal bar or some fruit and yogurt. For longer runs eat a larger snack or meal within one hour of finishing. Try an egg sandwich, cottage cheese with a baked potato or chicken with rice and vegetables.

meat, fish, eggs, low-fat dairy, beans and pulses, soy, protein powders and, to a lesser extent, green vegetables such as broccoli and spinach. A 100-gram chicken breast contains around 30 grams of protein, a 100-gram pot of cottage cheese contains 13 grams, two eggs offer 12 grams and a 100-gram tin of tuna contains around.

" To avoid energy dips and fatigue you need to replace glycogen stores."

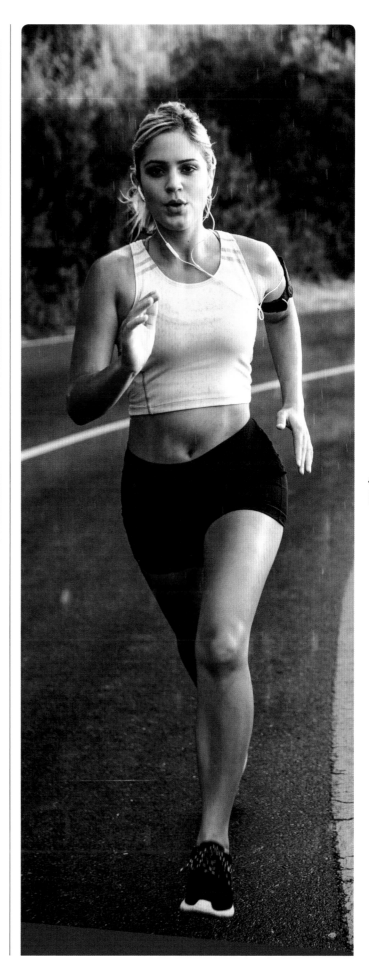

GLUTEN- AND DAIRY-FREE RUNNING

Analysing the benefits of cutting out wheat and dairy to improve your running.

It can be hard to differentiate diet fads from established advice, particularly when celebrity athletes have their individual cases in the spotlight. Paula Radcliffe found her gut problems were resolved when she removed foods to which she was diagnosed as intolerant from her diet. These included wheat (a source of gluten) and dairy. The paleo diet, known as the "caveman diet", which excludes all grains and dairy products, became popular among those seeking to improve both health and sports performance. But does this mean you should remove gluten and dairy from your diet? Will it improve your running or could it have negative effects on your energy, stamina and ability to recover from training and races?

Those with a medical diagnosis of coeliac disease, lactose intolerance or milk allergy have to exclude gluten or dairy from their diets. People who currently experience digestive health issues, such as loose bowels, abdominal discomfort, excessive flatulence or bloating, but have no medical diagnosis, may also see a benefit from excluding gluten and/or dairy. If your digestive health is currently good, you are less likely to see performance benefits from excluding these food types, although some people may. However, from a nutritional perspective, it can be beneficial to widen the variety of foods in your diet, so feel free to sometimes choose gluten- or dairy-free meals and snacks in place of your usual favourites.

KEEP IT NATURAL

It's perfectly possible to enjoy a healthy diet while excluding gluten and dairy products, so long as you make sure you choose largely natural, unprocessed foods, which provide a wide range of nutrients. The gluten-containing grains to be avoided – wheat, rye and barley – are good sources of B vitamins and magnesium, needed for energy production. This is one reason that pasta, made from wheat, is so popular with runners. Dairy foods such as milk, yogurt and cheese contain protein to help recovery from running and calcium to help maintain bone health. You will need to choose alternative sources of these nutrients. It's important to note that, while oats do not

contain gluten naturally, they are often grown in fields where contamination with gluten is a risk, so you will need to choose products that contain gluten-free oats.

RUNNING WITHOUT GLUTEN OR DAIRY IN YOUR DIET

The night before a long run or a race, the following choices will provide a good mix of starchy carbohydrates, a little protein and a range of vitamins and minerals:
- Risotto, made with rice, chicken or prawns and vegetables (no cheese)
- Corn or rice pasta with chicken, vegetables and tomato sauce (no cheese)
- Baked sweet potato and grilled chicken
- Quinoa, steamed and mixed with vegetables and fish, chicken or a hard-boiled egg
- New potato salad with poached salmon
- Sushi selection (six to eight pieces)

Choose one of these breakfasts, which should be eaten around two hours before you run:
- Gluten-free toast, with almond butter or mashed banana and honey
- Gluten-free porridge oats or quinoa flakes, with almond or soya milk
- Buckwheat pancakes with honey and berries

ALTERNATIVES POST-RUN

After your long run or race, you need to replenish your carbohydrate stores and take on board some protein to promote muscle recovery, ideally within 20 minutes. Most commercially available recovery drinks and bars use whey protein, which comes from milk. The best option is to make your own recovery drink, using an alternative protein powder, such as soya isolate, pea or hemp. These are available from health food shops or online. Blend the protein powder with fruit and non-dairy milk, such as coconut, almond, rice or soya. There are also gluten- and dairy-free recovery bars on the market. If you need to adopt a gluten- and dairy-free diet, follow these guidelines and you should be able to both run well and enjoy good health.

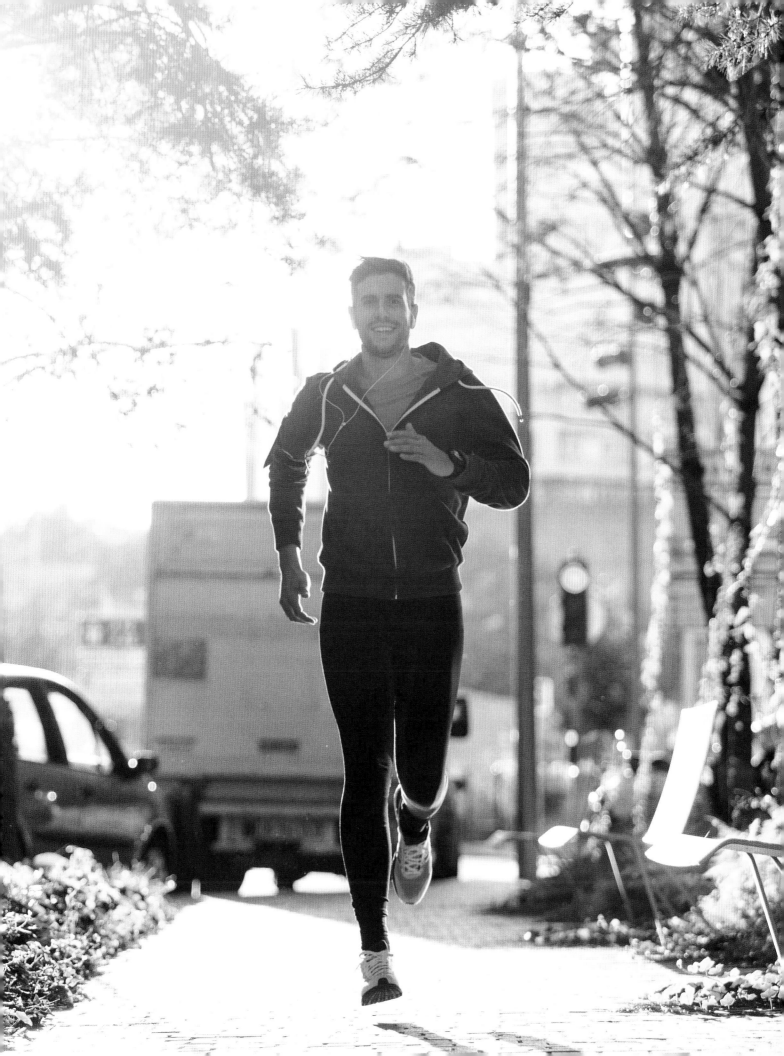

MANAGING WEIGHT

Many people take up running to lose weight, but end up actually putting on a few kilos. It doesn't have to be that way.

The single biggest mistake made by runners trying to lose weight is thinking they can eat whatever they want, simply because they run. This isn't always the case. It's easy to overestimate the amount of calorie-burning work you do in your run and just as easy to underestimate the calories in the biscuits or ice cream you consume after dinner as a reward. And even if your diet is generally good, you might still be overeating healthy food – all foods contain calories. Don't forget, however, that if you've just started running or if you're increasing your mileage, your weight gain may be the result of extra muscle.

BALANCING ACT

As a rule, you will burn between 80 and 100 calories for every ten minutes you run. So a 30-minute run would balance out the calories in one Mars bar. Also, it's common to feel hungry directly after a run. This is because your body's energy stores have been reduced and must be replaced. This is the time to eat food that's high in protein and has a small amount of carbohydrate (see pp.128–131). This will help to rebuild your muscles as well as replace the energy in those muscles (muscle glycogen) and in the liver (liver glycogen).

TAKE STOCK

Keeping a food and activity diary for a week is a good way to evaluate your habits. On one side of the page write down how long you have run for, how fast and (as accurately as you can) how many calories you have used each day. On the other side, write down what you had for breakfast, lunch, dinner, snacks and everything that you drank, noting how many calories you're consuming. Be honest – some people try to be extra good, but that will lead to a false reading if you keep up such a diet for only a week. Ensure you write down all your drinks – coffee and tea with sugar, sports drinks, fizzy drinks and fruit juices can add a significant number of calories. Be aware that an average woman needs about 2,000 calories a day while men need 2,500, but this will vary slightly depending on many factors, including age and activity level.

DON'T GIVE IN TO CRAVINGS

Treats are often used as a reward for hard work, but compare the calories with the effort needed to burn them off. Sugar cravings are your body's way of telling you that your blood sugar has dropped; it doesn't mean you have to stuff yourself with sugary food. Cravings last for about ten minutes so the best thing to do is distract yourself for those crucial minutes or go for a healthy option. Keep seeds or nuts to hand. If you run just before lunch or dinner, try to prepare your meals before you go out. This way you can ensure your food is ready as soon as you get in to prevent you from snacking before your meal. When you eat, use a smaller plate and avoid second helpings. It takes a few minutes for your brain to work out that your stomach is full, so drink some water and wait ten minutes before deciding if you need to eat more.

ALTERNATIVES TO SUGARY TREATS

• Instead of eating a full packet of M&M's, mix them up with sunflower and pumpkin seeds. This way you get your chocolate treat, but you eat less of it. The sunflower and pumpkin seeds are high in calcium and magnesium, minerals that are important for muscle function and bone strength.
• Add a scoop of protein powder, peanut butter or a seed mix to your smoothie, to increase the protein and mineral content.
• Instead of eating breakfast bars or cereal bars, try one of the bars on the market that's higher in protein.

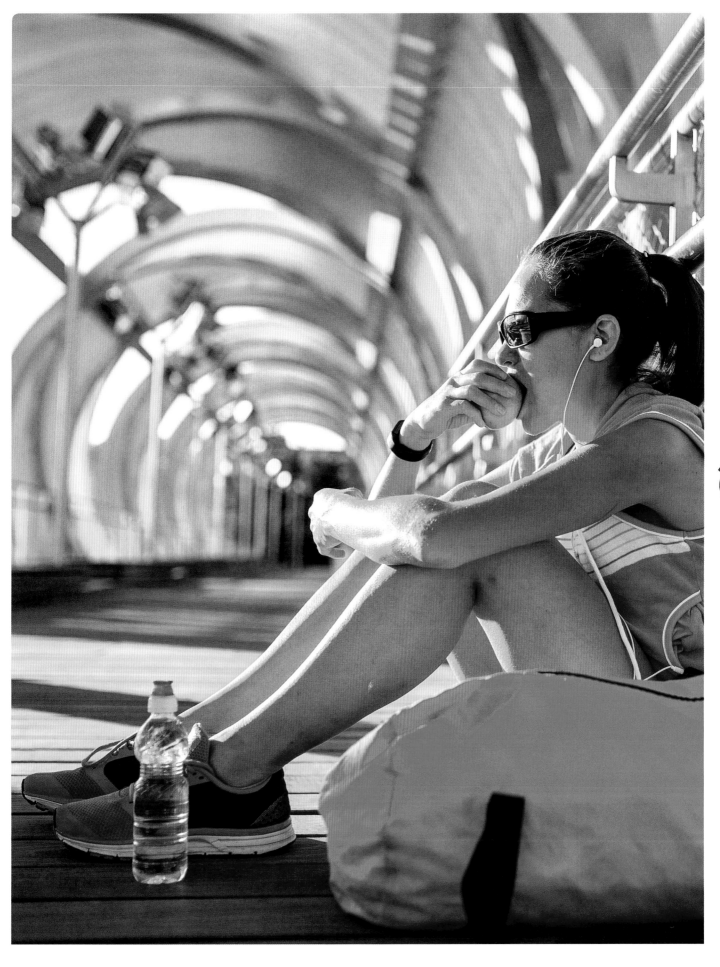

NUTRITION FOR LONG-DISTANCE RUNNING

Your diet is vital when you take on distances as long as a marathon.

As your weekly training mileage builds, you should plan how your diet will change. Not taking on board enough calories and nutrients is a classic mistake and one that could contribute to overtraining syndrome, causing your progress to stall. Training for a marathon with weight loss as your main goal is certainly not a good idea.

DON'T CURB CARBS AND BE PRO-PROTEIN
Carbohydrates are your main source of fuel for running, although you also obtain some energy from fat stores. The more miles you run, the higher your needs are. You'll need to obtain quickly absorbed carbs from energy gels and sports drinks during your long runs. Protein helps your muscles to recover from training and supports your immune system. Take on good-quality fats and keep treats to a minimum or you may gain weight – even if you're training for a marathon. For more details on general aspects of nutrition that apply to running, see pp.128–131.

glycogen stores are full on your big day. This doesn't mean eating more calories, but making starchy and sugary foods a bigger proportion of your diet than normal and cutting back on protein and fat. As well as eating bread, pasta, rice and potatoes, use fruit juices, fruit smoothies, jams, honey and energy bars to get your extra carbs. Make sure you have tried out your pre-race dinner the night before one of your long runs, and keep it low in fat, fibre and spices to prevent stomach problems. Try to eat no later than 7 pm.

RACE DAY NUTRITION
Have a tried-and-tested breakfast at least two hours before a marathon. This might be porridge and banana or white toast and jam or a bagel with honey. But a simple fruit smoothie or sports drink may be all you can manage. Drink around 500 ml of water in the hour or two before the start, factoring in a last toilet visit. Finally, take an energy gel and a little water or a few sips of sports drink ten to 15 minutes before you start the race.

RUNNING MENU

PRE-RUN – choose carbs that release energy quickly and contain less fibre.
EVENING RUNS – white bread or bagels, white rice or pasta, rice cakes or an energy bar are all good examples of snacks.
BREAFAST RUN – banana or diluted fruit juice for a hard session such as hills, intervals or tempo. On a slower-paced short run, you may prefer not to eat or drink anything. Always eat a good quality breakfast every day, whether you have a run or not.

THE WEEK BEFORE YOUR RACE
As you start your taper, you should reduce the amount of carbohydrate in your diet in line with your reduced mileage or you risk weight gain. Three days before your marathon, start the carbohydrate-loading process to ensure your

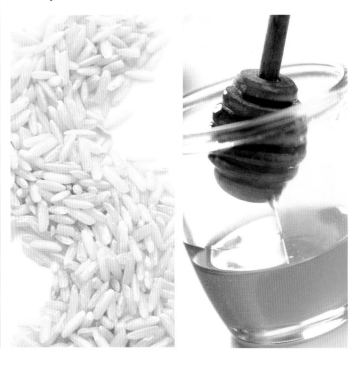

During the race, use the fuelling and hydration strategy that you have practised. Check beforehand where sports drinks will be found on the course or carry your own gels. Know where the water points will be. Don't leave it more than an hour before the first time you take on some energy replenishment. Keep yourself well hydrated with water, but use your thirst as a guide. Drinking too much dilutes the sodium levels in your blood and can result in a dangerous medical condition called hyponatraemia. Symptoms include nausea and vomiting, confusion, headaches and, in severe cases, loss of consciousness and coma.

MARATHON RACE RECOVERY

Make sure you have access to your favourite recovery product and use it within 20 minutes of finishing. Drink 500 ml to a litre of water in the first hour after the race and keep drinking until your urine is pale. Enjoy your post-run meal within two hours, but make sure it contains some carbs, protein and vegetables. Then have a further snack or recovery drink about two hours later, to prevent an energy crash. If you're struggling to eat solid foods, flavoured milk or fruit yogurt are good options.

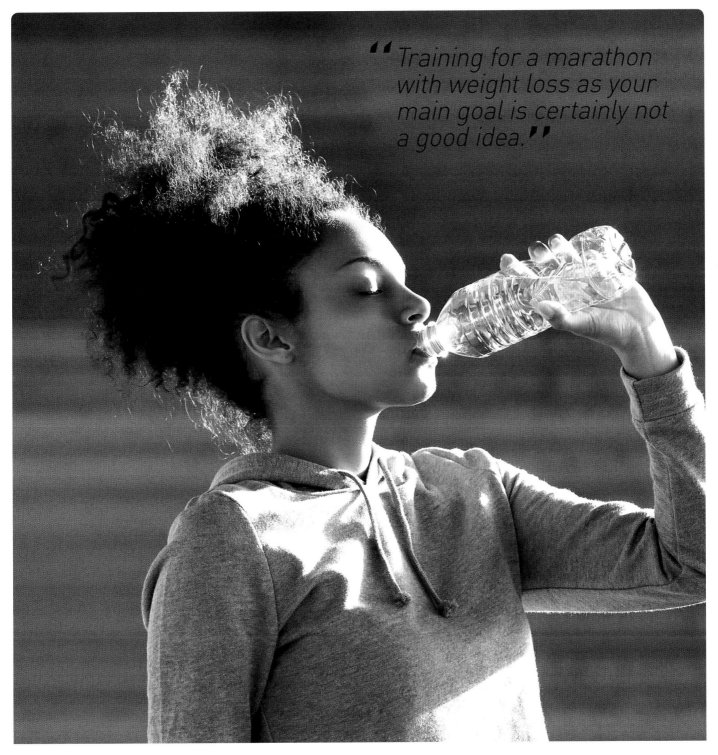

" Training for a marathon with weight loss as your main goal is certainly not a good idea. "

ADVICE ON SUPPLEMENTS

Taking a gel or energy drink one a long run can boost your performance.

Taking gels helps to replace your carbohydrate stores, known as glycogen, which you use to create energy as you run. Gels help to maintain energy levels and enable you to run for longer, but should only be used when you will be running for an hour or more. This is because your muscles store enough glycogen to fuel your running up to this time. Energy gels, in the form of semi-liquid goo in a packet, provide you with a concentrated burst of energy. Simply tear open and swallow while running.

The main ingredient in a gel is carbohydrate. This could be either the simple sugars glucose and fructose or maltodextrin, a starch manufactured from glucose. Most gels contain a combination of carbohydrate types. This is because glucose and fructose are carried into your bloodstream by different biochemical mechanisms. Studies have shown you cannot absorb more than 60 grams of glucose per hour, but adding fructose increases total sugar absorption to around 90 grams, enabling more energy to be created. Gels also contain some water, electrolyte minerals such as sodium and potassium, plus flavouring and preservatives. They may also contain caffeine, as this has been shown to benefit performance. Some gels are more diluted and easier to swallow than others. Most gels need to be washed down with water or may not be absorbed into your bloodstream quickly enough. Always check the label and stay well hydrated as you run.

GEL TEST

Experiment with different brands to see which you prefer and do this well before race day to avoid nasty digestive surprises. You can consume up to 30 grams of glucose or maltodextrin, or up to 45 grams of glucose-fructose mix per half hour of running. That's equivalent to two or three gels per hour, depending on the brand's formulation. It's best not to wait until you have been running for an hour before taking your first gel – even though it is quickly absorbed, the effect isn't instant. Try your first gel 30 to 40 minutes into your run and experiment to work out how often you need to take a gel during long runs.

Some people experience stomach cramps, tummy upsets or nausea from gels. This may be a difficulty tolerating fructose, in which case it's worth trying a brand that contains only glucose or maltodextrin. It could be problems with the caffeine in some gels or simply a sensitive stomach. Never try a new gel on race day!

ENERGY DRINKS

For shorter runs, stick to water or low-calorie electrolyte drinks, as hydration is your priority. Energy drinks, like gels, help to replace glycogen stores and their primary ingredient will be carbohydrate together with electrolyte minerals. They also give you the water you need.

Choose an energy drink that has been formulated for sport, with a concentration of 6–9 grams of carbohydrate per 100 grams of fluid. This will be shown on the label. Drinks such as fruit juice or highly caffeinated "energy" products such as Red Bull are too highly concentrated for use during exercise. They take longer to empty from your stomach and may cause discomfort, as well as failing to refuel you as quickly as sports drinks. Fruit juice may work for you if it's well diluted.

SHAKEN OR STIRRED

Sports drinks come ready mixed in a 500 ml or 750 ml bottle or as a powder that you mix into water and carry in a drinking bottle. It may be easier start with sachets rather than tubs, to ensure you're using the correct amount of powder. This will vary by brand, but it's likely to be one sachet with 400 to 500 ml of water. Aim to drink at least half a litre of energy drink per hour – more on a hot day. Take only several sips at regular intervals to avoid stomach problems. Practise using in training, to make sure you can tolerate your brand for race day.

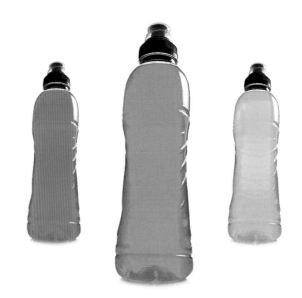

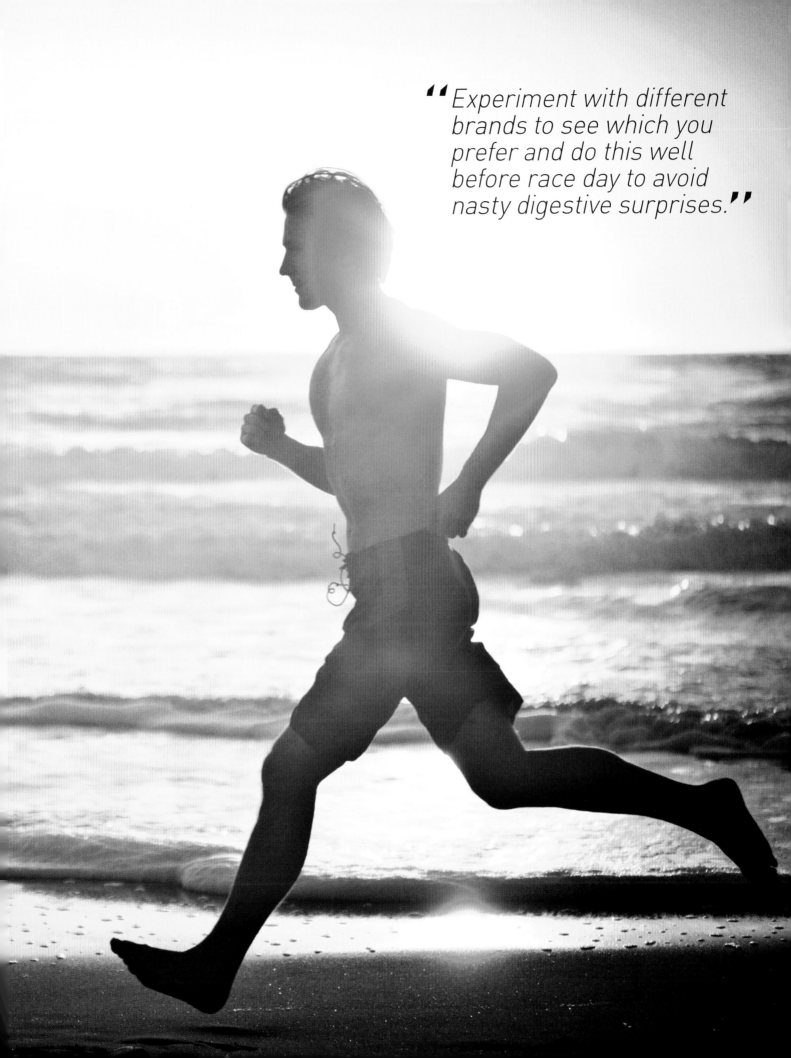

"Experiment with different brands to see which you prefer and do this well before race day to avoid nasty digestive surprises."

RECOVERY NUTRITION

Get your post-run snack just right.

You've just finished a hard run and feel shattered, but before you put your feet up, you need to refuel your tired muscles. The quicker you consume food after a run, the quicker your body will recover. The ideal post-training snack should supply carbohydrate to replenish depleted glycogen stores, as well as protein to repair and rebuild the muscles. Here are some top foods for recovery from running.

BLACKBERRIES

Avoid the risk of post-race colds by eating blackberries. Their high levels of natural phenolic acids help kill viruses and fight infections. Just 15 berries provide around one third of the vitamin C you need each day, as well as half the vitamin E (which helps relieve post-run soreness).

RAISINS

Raisins are a concentrated source of carbohydrate, which makes for a useful post-run snack when you need a quick energy boost. They are also a rich source of fibre, potassium, and antioxidant vitamins and minerals.

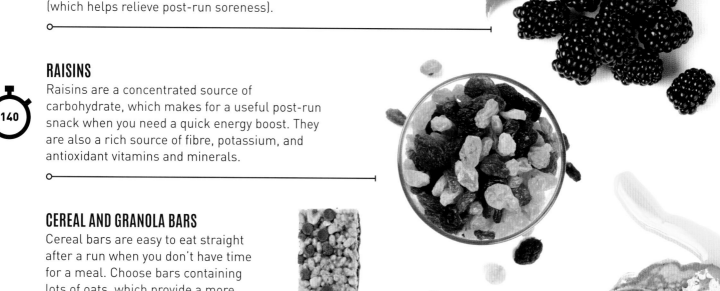

CEREAL AND GRANOLA BARS

Cereal bars are easy to eat straight after a run when you don't have time for a meal. Choose bars containing lots of oats, which provide a more sustained energy boost, as well as a little more protein than other cereals. Most bars supply around 90 to 130 calories and less than 5g fat, which makes them quick to digest and a healthier alternative to biscuits.

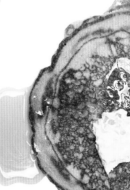

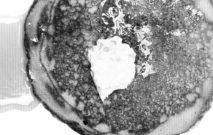

PANCAKES

Make your own or buy ready-made pancakes for a high-carb post-run snack. Two pancakes provide about 200 calories and 30g of carbohydrate to refuel depleted muscles. They also supply 5-7g protein, which accelerates glycogen storage and rebuilds muscle cells. Top with a little honey or, for added vitamins, a tablespoon of stewed apples.

BAKED BEANS

Great for soluble fibre (which helps lower blood sugar and cholesterol levels), baked beans also give you 10g protein per 200g serving – about the same as a large slice (40g) of cheese. Beans are also rich in iron, essential for transporting oxygen around the body, as well as B vitamins, zinc and magnesium. Eat on toast, with a baked potato or, if you absolutely must, straight from the can!

FLAVOURED MILK

Milk's high protein and carbohydrate content helps refuel exhausted muscles. A 2008 study by researchers at Northumbria University found that athletes who drank 500ml of semi-skimmed milk or chocolate milk immediately after training had less muscle soreness and more rapid muscle recovery than those using commercial sports drinks or water.

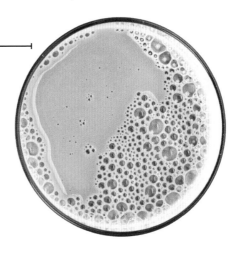

NUTS

All nuts are a good source of protein, fibre, heart-protective vitamin E and B vitamins (which help release energy from food). They not only promote muscle recovery after a run, but can also help you shed pounds. A study from Harvard Medical School found that people who ate nuts as part of a Mediterranean diet lost more weight and kept it off longer than those who followed a traditional low-fat diet.

RICE CAKES WITH PEANUT BUTTER

Plain rice cakes can provide a quick energy boost after a run, but eating them with a little peanut butter is even better. This combination provides the perfect ratio of carbs to protein (4:1) for speedy glycogen refuelling and muscle repair. Peanut butter also provides protein, fibre and vitamin E.

YOGHURT

Fruit yoghurt contains carbohydrate (lactose and sucrose) and protein in a 4:1 ratio. According to a study at the University of Texas, this nutrient ratio accelerates post-exercise refuelling, which means faster recovery and muscles that feel less sore the next day. Yoghurt is also rich in bone-building calcium.

SIMPLE SUPERFOODS

Keep healthy eating simple with these everyday superfoods.

You don't need to spend a fortune on berries handpicked in the middle of the Amazon Rainforest to make sure you're getting your quota of superfoods. These are all super-nutritious, super-cheap and super-easy to find – forget hunting down a far-out health food store, you'll find this list in your local supermarket.

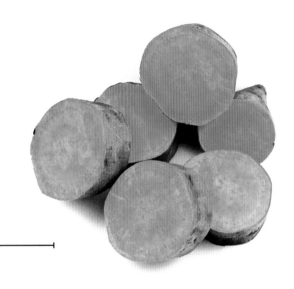

SWEET POTATOES
Despite their name, sweet potatoes aren't potatoes at all – they aren't even related! Originally from Central America, they are a nutritious vegetable with a low GI (glycaemic index), meaning they provide a gradual release of energy. They also contain vitamin C for a strong immune system; magnesium, which helps the body use energy from food; and manganese, important for healthy bones and joints.

WATERCRESS
Watercress is packed with vitamins A, C and E for healthy skin and a strong immune system, plus calcium and vitamin K, important for blood clotting and bone strength. It also contains folic acid and iron, both crucial to build healthy red blood cells and needed to transport oxygen to working muscle cells. The vitamin C in watercress boosts the absorption of its iron content, too. It also contains lutein, beta-carotene and flavonoids which, along with vitamins C and E, help protect your body's cells from the potentially damaging effects of free radicals.

WHOLEGRAIN CEREAL
Any variety will do, providing it's labelled "wholegrain". A study found that, compared with a commercial sports drink, a bowl of wholegrain cereal and skimmed milk was at least as good at promoting muscle refuelling and recovery. The cereal helped replenish glycogen (carbohydrate stores) in muscles just as well as the carbohydrate-containing sports drink. Fortified breakfast cereals also provide useful amounts of B vitamins, which allow the body to release energy from food, and iron to help prevent energy-sapping anaemia.

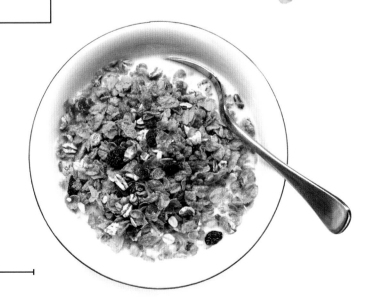

BEETROOT

Beetroot brims with folic acid, needed for cell division and building healthy red blood cells, which transport oxygen to help fuel your muscles. Beetroot has been ranked among the top ten most powerful vegetable sources of antioxidants, thanks to its content of phenolics and betacyanin. Antioxidants help to protect body cells from the potentially damaging effects of free radicals, which are increased during exercise. Drinking two large glasses of beetroot juice a day could help you exercise for 16 per cent longer at the same intensity, according to a small study in the *Journal Of Applied Physiology*.

SALMON

Salmon's benefits lie in its supply of muscle-restoring protein, healthy fats, and key vitamins and minerals. Take vitamin D – as well as being important for a healthy immune system, it allows the body to absorb calcium. Salmon is one of the few good food sources – an average portion of cooked salmon (100g) provides more than 100 per cent of the recommended daily allowance (RDA). Salmon also supplies omega-3 fatty acids, known for helping to keep the heart and joints healthy.

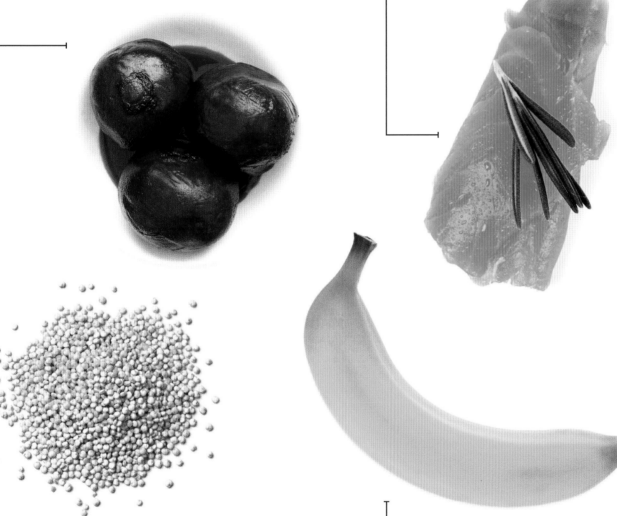

143

QUINOA

Quinoa contains twice as much protein as rice. As well as supporting post-running muscle recovery, protein helps you feel fuller for longer, making it easier to keep calorie intake – and weight – in check. Quinoa also brims with energy-giving carbohydrates, which are slowly released to provide a steady fuel supply to exercising or refuelling muscles. More good news is that it supplies key minerals, such as iron, bone-friendly magnesium, zinc (for a strong immune system) and potassium (essential for muscle contraction and keeping the body hydrated), along with folic acid, needed to enable the body to use protein for repair and to prevent anaemia.

BANANAS

Packed with energy-giving carbohydrate, a medium banana contains around 95 calories. They also have a low GI, meaning their energy is released in a slow and sustained way, ideal for fuelling your running and aiding post-run muscle recovery. One banana counts as one of your recommended five or more portions of fruit and vegetables a day, and therefore brims with cell- and immunity-protecting antioxidants, including vitamin C.

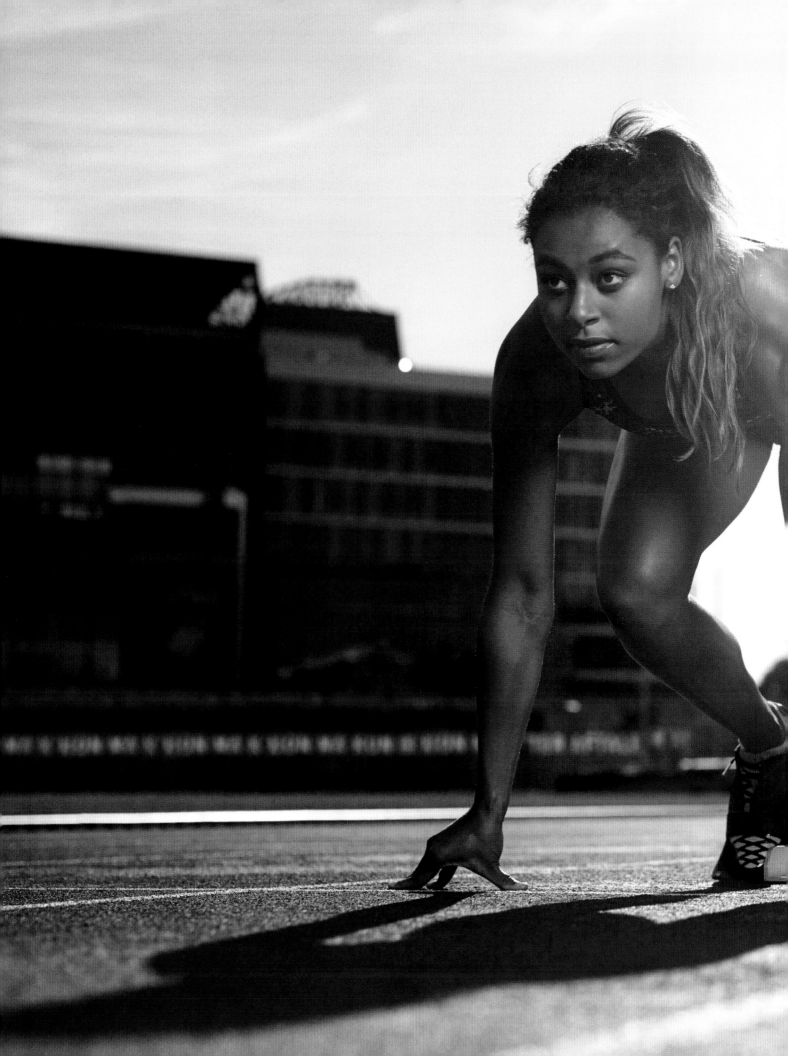

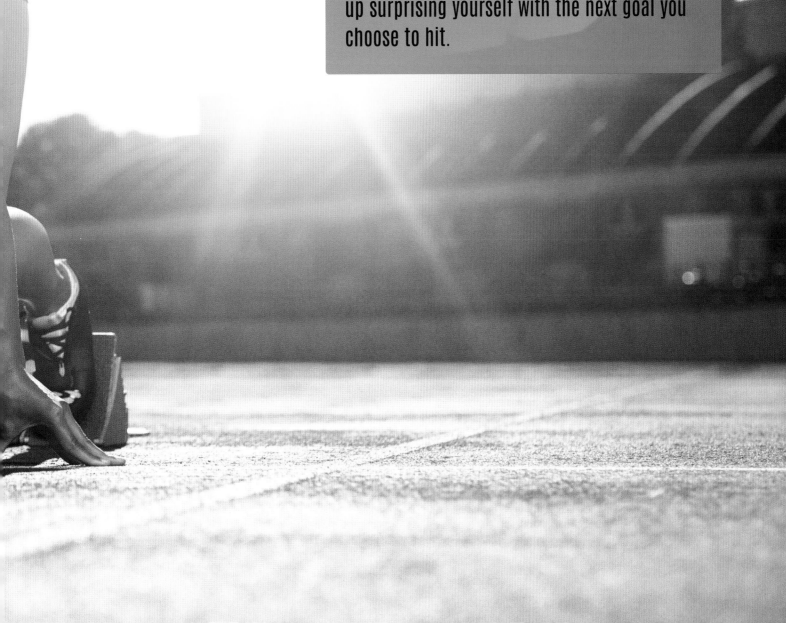

BECOMING A PRO

Tips from the experts, athlete interviews and a glimpse at the world of the elite runners. Even if you never plan to do more than a few circuits of your local park, you'll find something to interest you and you may end up surprising yourself with the next goal you choose to hit.

MAKE THE DISTANCE SAFELY

Around 79 per cent of runners suffer from injury each year, so it pays to be smart when it comes to distance running.

When you get a few shorter races under your belt, it's natural to want to step up to a half-marathon, a marathon or maybe even an ultra. However, conquering distance running is about much more than just increasing your mileage.

"People often make the mistake of immediately increasing distance and just focusing on that," said running coach Keith Anderson. "Quite often that results in injury, even in really good runners. Going up in distance needs careful thought and respect to make sure you don't end up with an overuse injury." Don't increase your total weekly mileage by more than 10 per cent. If you keep a training diary you can look back at your sessions and find a pattern between good or bad runs and other lifestyle factors, such as sleep, rest and nutrition.

KEEP AN EYE ON YOUR FEET
The style you use when you run can affect whether or not you get injured, especially when you're incrementing distance. "Everything stems from the feet but we don't pay enough attention to this, which can have harsh consequences in the long term," said Pilates instructor and personal trainer Kate McTaggart. "If you're pressing more weight through one foot than the other, you're going to get all sorts of imbalances. Or if you have tight glutes and your inner thighs are too weak to keep your feet straight when you run, with every step you take you are accentuating that imbalance every time. This can cause knee and hip issues." Visit a physiotherapist or running coach and seek advice on your technique and never increase distance and intensity together.

FOLLOW A STRUCTURED PLAN
A typical week can include one long run, a threshold session and another slightly more challenging run on an undulating surface at a higher intensity. You don't need to do more than one long run per week, so long as you are consistent with doing that training every week. Be patient. Becoming a good distance runner can take time, even if you are fit through other sports. You have got to give it time

to get your tendons and ligaments conditioned. Endurance is borne out by many weeks and months, if not years, of solid training.

Ensure you have enough time to train for an event. Going from 10K to a half-marathon is logical, given up to four months of training. Give yourself something more like six months in order to get up to marathon standard, to gradually layer on the long runs and make the body better conditioned and stronger. Around six months is also a realistic timeframe for anyone going from a marathon to an ultra. Use conditioning work for the muscles involved in the repetition of the foot hitting the ground repeatedly.

Rotate two pairs of running shoes – they can be the same shoes, but an older and a newer pair will mean you can use the newer shoes for harder sessions and the older pair for recovery runs or sessions on more forgiving surfaces like grass. Anderson said not to use thin, lightweight shoes and spikes. "Some people go to a running track and pound around on spikes that are five years old and the inside lane is like concrete as so many people have run over it. Shoes must be in good condition."

STRENGTH AND CONDITIONING
"I try to lift fairly heavy weights so I will do eight to 10 reps of squats, deadlifts, lunges and also upper body like chest press," said marathon runner Tracy McCartney. "I also do lots of core work like the plank and Russian twists. I do three sessions of strength training per week." If you haven't done any strength work before, then start with circuit training-style strength work, for which you don't need a gym. Try squats, lunges and step-ups instead.

" I'm very relaxed. I don't get anxious about my running. I try to enjoy it."

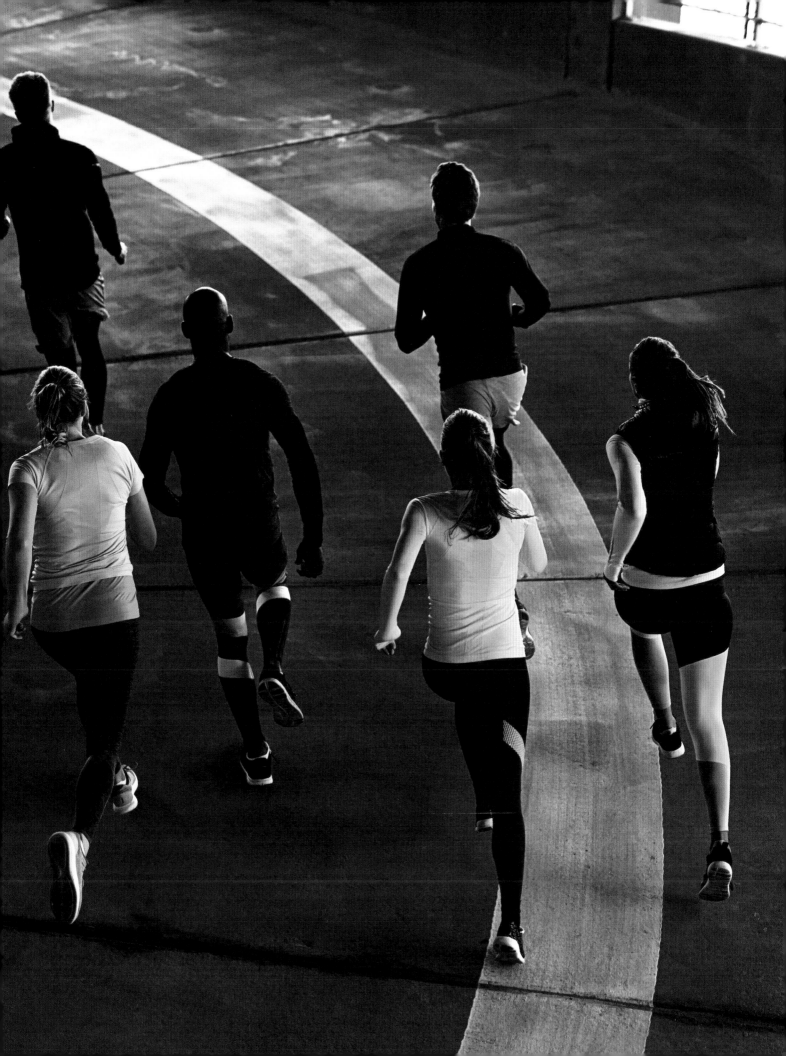

Do remember to include recovery weeks in your training. Have an easier fourth or fifth week to allow your body to recover from the increase in mileage, where you can temporarily cut back on mileage and perhaps have an extra rest day. "If you just keep adding miles the body doesn't get a chance to adapt," said Anderson. "It's like working under pressure – you get it done but when you lie on the beach you realise how shattered you are – similarly, when you get to the end of the taper or end of the training cycle, you realise that the niggle you've had is getting worse. Your body has to be able to cope and adapt to the workload."

DON'T BE A FUEL FOOL

The less fat you carry, the easier you will find running. When you run, approximately three-and-a-half times your body weight is absorbed through the joints, so even losing 1.3 kg could reduce the impact by almost 5 kg and make running easier. But don't confuse body fat with muscle – you may stay at the same weight if you have gained muscle but your body composition will have improved, as you'll have more muscle and less body fat.

Avoid strict dieting – focus on the quality of your food and you will probably lose a few pounds anyway. For more details on nutrition, see chapter 4, beginning p.126. "You need to make sure you are feeding the engine and not trying to do anything faddy," said Anderson. "You are really trying to look after your energy reserves and allow for growth and repair after a training session."

Have a recovery drink after a long run. High quality carbohydrates and protein immediately after a long run will give your body the ability to recover. If you don't feel like eating straight away, a recovery drink may be the answer. You can read more about this on pp.136–137. Don't end up in a state where you don't replenish after harder sessions. You need to be on top form for your next session. If you ignore that principle, you end up running on 75 per cent fuel and the next time it's 50 per cent and that will just drag you down.

Work on mental strength, as long distances, particularly over the marathon format, are fought in your head. Positive mental tactics will override anything. During training, practise mental tactics, visualise feeling good. When you start feeling rubbish, tell yourself you are feeling good.

MAKE RUNNING FUN

When you are putting yourself under pressure to go out and complete a long run, it can become a chore. Remember you've chosen to do it because you want to and not because you have to. Tracy McCartney attributed her success as a distance runner to her enjoyment of it. "I'm very relaxed. I don't get anxious about my running. I try to enjoy it and I also try to run in places that I love. I go on holiday to Cornwall and Devon in the UK and get as many runs as I possibly can across the coastline. I do races that I enjoy."

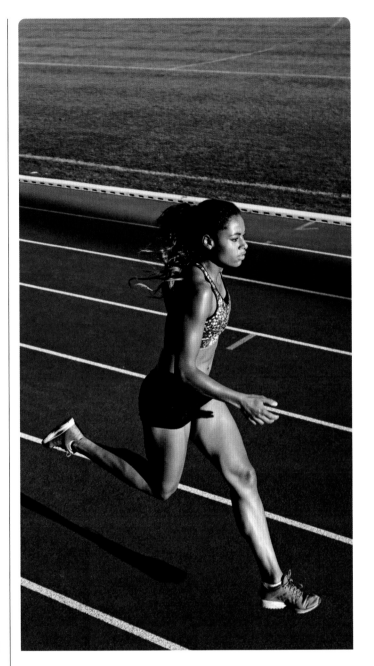

"Keep a training log to see how much you're doing because consistency is the biggest key for results."

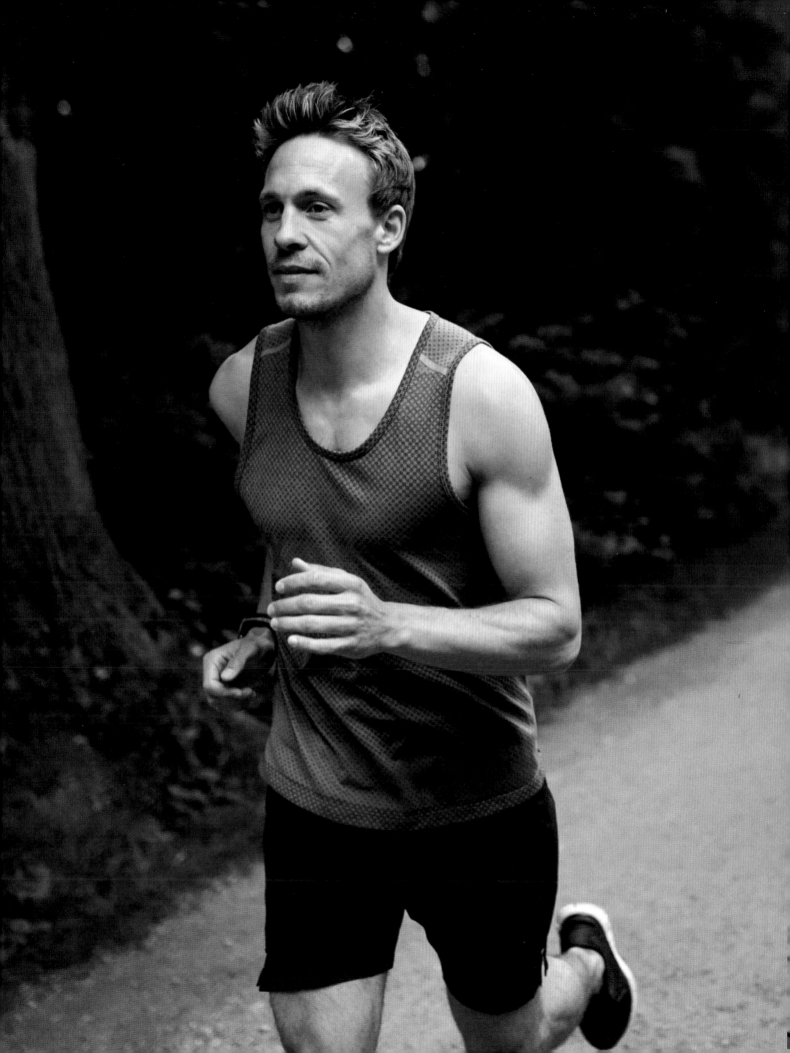

LEADER OF THE PACK

Competing against yourself is great, but you need to cope when you're fighting for a podium place.

Some people are not too sure how to react the first time they reach the winners' podium. On the one hand, reaching the prizes – or just moving into a Top 10 position – is a brilliant feeling. You may find you like this feeling and you want to keep aiming high – you have raised your performance bar without even realising it. You need to know how to stay on top and get used to being at the sharp end.

It can be easy to become distracted by what other runners find successful while training. During a race, it's even harder to run for yourself, as your success in placing high could depend to an extent on being aware of the other runners around you and responding to their tactics. But it's important that you still know how you tick: what is the fastest pace you can hold to the finish, what does that feel like and what will it take to get you there? This will often mean having the confidence to do things differently to runners around you and sometimes accepting that they are simply faster than you at the moment, but in the long-term you'll run better this way.

CALL IN THE COACH

Ask for professional help. You are not looking for someone to completely tear up your training schedule and give you a totally new approach – after all, you have already shown that you can run fast. You are looking for someone who understands how you think, how you like to train and the other pressures on your life. Most importantly, you're looking for a coach who can offer you the emotional and psychological support you'll need to stay at the front end of the race. A good coach will keep you calm when you're panicked by other people's fitness levels or when you want to throw your race plan out of the window and pelt off at a stupid pace straight from the gun. They will review each race and session so you learn and move forwards. If you're not already part of a club, joining one and getting coaching support (as well as other fast runners to train with) is a brilliant place to start.

Training works better when it is specifically tailored to an event, so choose one you want to be really good at. You might decide you want to be great at flat 5K races or you want to excel at lumpy off-road courses. Just choose your area of focus and put everything into that.

This also applies to your race planning. Choose a few

A-races to aim for and plan everything else around those. Work with your coach to decide how you'll approach each event so that you're not constantly asking too much of your body. Save your hard efforts for those key events.

LOOK AROUND YOU

"Great camaraderie." Time and time again you'll hear this cited as one of the brilliant things about the running community. But once you are competing for a race place rather than just against yourself, you will need to think slightly differently. You'll need to become aware of the other racers who have entered your chosen event, how they usually run, and their previous finish times. You'll need to be prepared to pick them off as you run through the field. In local races or those you compete in regularly, you'll get to know a few names and faces who will always be in the Top 20. Make use of this knowledge to determine your own goals – and don't forget to be as friendly and supportive as ever over the finish line.

Find running partners who challenge you. That doesn't mean ditching lifelong running buddies, but making sure you do the intense sessions with runners who are slightly faster than you are. It might be intimidating at first, but once you find the right group of people to train with, you'll find your speed comes on.

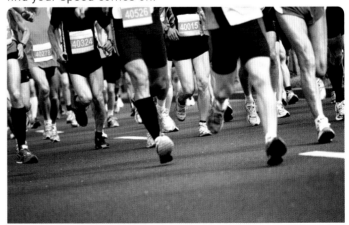

" Have the confidence to do things differently to runners around you. "

150

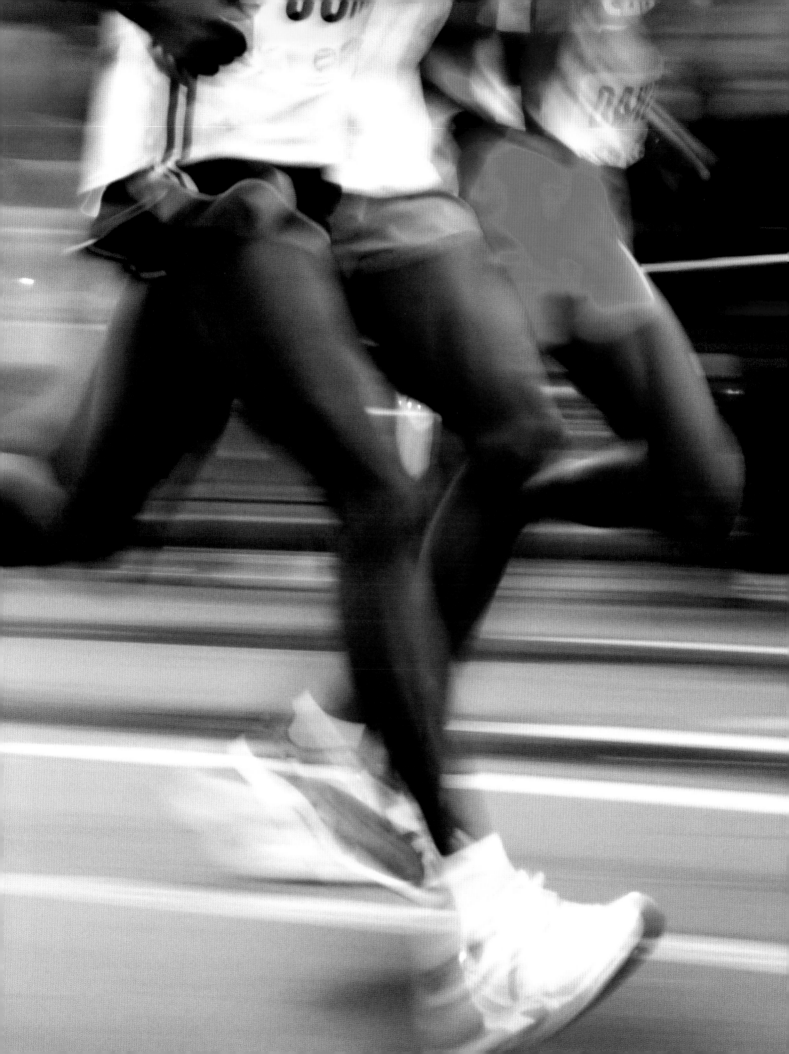

REAL EXPERIENCE: NUTRITION

Runners talk about how crucial it is to get it right when it comes to fuelling.

Christina Macdonald is the editor-in-chief of Women's Running. She struggled with her running when her dieting became too extreme and only injury forced her to get those bad eating habits under control.

"I got into running for weight loss. As I built up my stamina and was able to run further, the weight began to fall off. I had never felt slimmer and fitter. I became addicted to the buzz of running, so I would take to the treadmill and run for an hour most days. People began to express concern, commenting about my looking pale, drawn and tired. I didn't want to hear them.

152

"I managed to lose 8 kg in three months, but I noticed myself starting to change. My energy levels had dipped. Despite going to bed early, I couldn't shift the black rings around my eyes. I was in peak condition, yet I was permanently knackered. Then my periods stopped altogether. I knew I couldn't be pregnant; it was just that I was clearly underweight for my body type."

ADDICTED TO DIETING

"I survived on just 900 calories daily and ran five or six miles most days until I got a stress fracture that forced me to take a break from running for six weeks. I managed to get my life back and I put on 3 kg. It felt very good to be back in control. My running has significantly improved too. I've been able to complete five half-marathons, one marathon and many 10K races.

"My favourite running foods for energy now include fruit bread, pasta, hummus and salad. And my post-run snacks include jacket potatoes, mackerel on toast with veggies or poached salmon with rice and veggies. Where weight loss is concerned, there simply are no shortcuts. Only a sensible training plan and a healthy approach to food will do."

" Since resuming normal eating habits, my running has significantly improved."

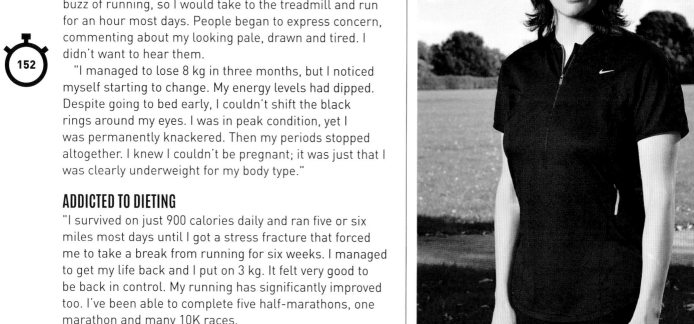

through my running history. I told him I thought I was doing too much running because I was tired all the time. He stopped me and asked about my diet.

"I've battled with my weight all my life and have always counted the calories daily. I broke down what I ate. I was consuming 1,750 calories a day, adding 100 calories per mile on run days, but the weight was still going on. I would often skip breakfast on non-run days, then have fruit for the rest of the day, maybe a salad for lunch, and finish with a sensible dinner of meat and vegetables. At weekends I binged on biscuits and sweet things, but come Monday, I was back on the diet. Nick explained that my body had gone into starvation mode and my metabolism had slowed down. I needed to eat more to lose weight.

"Within days my energy levels were up. I had more substantial breakfasts of wholemeal bread and peanut butter, cereal or porridge. I snacked on oatcakes and rice cakes and sipped on sports drinks. I had bigger lunches, with pasta and rice and I stopped counting calories."

QUALITY TRAINING

"The biggest difference I noticed was at the start of my long runs. Previously, in the first four miles, I felt tight, stiff and my heart rate would race. Since I started eating well and fuelling properly, I can head out of the door and feel normal from mile one. By eating during long runs and fuelling properly, I finish much fresher and the following day I can get straight back into it, so the quality and intensity of my sessions has improved too. To sum up my new philosophy, it's 'Eat to run, don't run to eat.'"

153

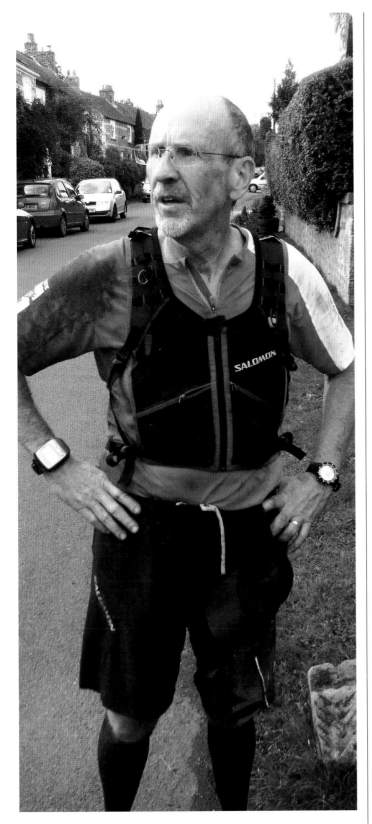

Seasoned runner Gary Tebbutt was low on energy and suffering during his long runs, until he overhauled his fuelling.

"I trained for an ultra-marathon as a seasoned marathon runner who wanted a new challenge. At the start of the programme, I sat down with coach Nick Anderson to go

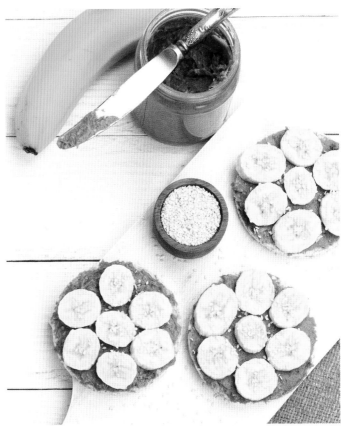

REAL EXPERIENCE: NELL MCANDREW AT THE LONDON MARATHON

In 2012, at the age of 38, Nell McAndrew secured her fastest time and never felt fitter.

Model-turned-marathon-runner Nell McAndrew ran London for the first time in 2003, finishing in an impressive 3:22:29. In 2012 she posted a personal best of 2:54:39, through hard work and dedication. Even with two young children, she continued to run.

154

"I wanted to try to beat my previous time, so I started Googling sub three-hour marathon discussions. I already had a book called Marathon Running by Richard Nerurkar so I thought I should just piece bits of advice together, mixing and matching to create a training programme. I knew I would have to increase my mileage to be in with a chance. Doing more long runs in training definitely made a difference.

"I must admit that, at times, it was hard to keep my motivation going – winter training is not always that appealing. But I felt that my running was gradually improving. I felt more efficient and faster, and I began to recover better after each run. Fitting in training around being a mum and my career was hard. Having a training plan helped, because I'd look at it and think: 'Right, that's what I have to do tomorrow,' and I'd just add it to my to-do list without thinking about it. I'd sometimes have to move days around and do my long run on a Saturday if it worked better around family commitments."

EARLY TRAINING RUNS

"I'd sometimes get up early and get one short run done and out of the way. I also ran on my way to school in the afternoon, as that meant I was using my time more efficiently. Instead of getting the tube or a taxi home, I ran home with my backpack, because I knew I had to do a long run that day. On weekends, if we were going for a family swim, I'd run to the swimming pool and get my husband and son to meet me there. I'd just set off 15 minutes earlier.

"I've always loved my food, probably because I exercise a lot. That's kept me eating better than I would have done as a model, because you can't exercise on fresh air or rubbish. My breakfast is usually natural yogurt with strawberries, or porridge with fruit; for lunch I will have one or two tins of mackerel with granary bread; mid-afternoon I snack on celery, carrots and cucumber; and dinner is normally a spinach omelette with beans or pasta with tomatoes, courgettes, mushrooms, pepper, chilli and garlic. I also take an iron supplement and snack on almonds, cashews, bananas or protein bars.

"On the day of the marathon itself, I started off too fast, but I realised my mistake straight away and slowed down. But overall I felt really comfortable. Nutrition was key – I sipped an SiS carbohydrate powder diluted with water, then threw away my bottle when it ran out. I'd love to run the Virgin London Marathon when I'm 80! Not walk it – I'd want to at least be able to jog it and keep going, because to me that's what it's all about."

FINDING TIME TO TRAIN

- Plan your day the night before and work out when you'll have time to run.
- Break sessions up into two shorter runs if you don't have time for one long exercise session.
- Remember, the cumulative effect of running is beneficial too. Completing two short runs is just as good as one longer run.
- Encourage friends to run with you so you can enlist their support. Even if they aren't training for a marathon, they can join you on part of your long run to break it up and take your mind off the time.

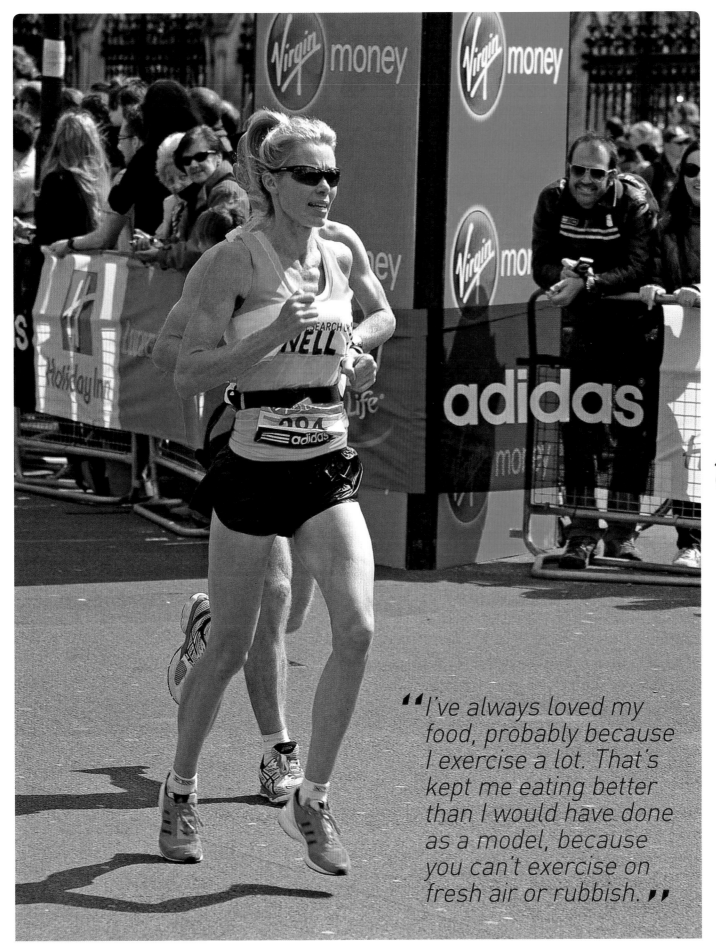

"I've always loved my food, probably because I exercise a lot. That's kept me eating better than I would have done as a model, because you can't exercise on fresh air or rubbish."

REAL EXPERIENCE: TRAILS

Runners who choose the trails over road running every time have a variety of reasons, from stress relief to a love of mud.

Fiona Salt, 37, lives in Adlington, Lancashire, UK, and has been trail running on the West Pennine moors for two years. She does three trail runs a week of between four and eight miles.

"The beautiful scenery and the sounds of nature enable me to switch off from life's distractions. I get really immersed in a trail run, whereas on roads it's all about chasing a time, waiting for traffic lights and dodging teenagers at the bus stop. I have a hectic life, teaching A-level English full-time and bringing up two young children. Running is my 'me time' and trail running has the bonus of literally getting me away from it all. I started running to ease postnatal depression and it really did help."

IMPROVING FITNESS

"My ankles cope with hills better than before and my core muscles are stronger – I think all the uneven ground of trail running really strengthens those two areas. Running with a club motivates me on a cold, rainy day. Also, I wouldn't be so adventurous without them in terms of where I go. I'm pretty directionally challenged, so if I headed off into deep trail territory without them leading the way, I'd probably end up being shot at in a farmer's field."

" Trail running makes me appreciate things more, gives me freedom and makes me happy."

Ross Lawrie trail runs in Scotland and has also run in the Lake District. He has completed the D33 Ultra, a 33-mile race beginning and ending in Aberdeen.

"I grew up in the countryside, so this plays a big factor in what draws me to spending time outdoors, enjoying time on the hills, as I did as a child. Trail running has less impact on your body than road running. I have been running barefoot-style for about three years and I feel

as though I can sense and connect more directly to my environment. I find that I can release any stresses in day-to-day life, when I plug myself in and connect with the Earth. Running barefoot also reminds me of the times when I ran as a kid, exploring new places."

RELAXATION

"I often find myself switching off into a natural meditative state of mind. This is a fantastic way to end a stressful day or week of work, leaving me refreshed and buzzing for more. Trail running also showed me that I could run distances that I initially thought were unachievable."

TRAINING BENEFITS

"Shorter distances can be just as much of a workout on the body because of the undulating and rough terrain that you may need to cover. Hill sessions and serious inclines are easier to find on trails and the rough ground will also offer a strong workout to your whole body.

"I love food but I now look at it as a necessary fuel that my body requires to perform well. This has introduced me to newer food groups and I now buy more of my usual healthier foods, rather than getting the same old same old for lunch. Regular healthy snacks throughout the day are important and you should also drink plenty of water.

"My dream trails would be the Everest Marathon and the Ultra Caballo Blanco in Mexico."

EXTREME TRAILS

Jonathan Mackintosh, Scotland: "I have no great aversion to road running, but I would always choose a trail run over a road run, regardless of the weather conditions. Trail running offers me greater freedom and lets me reconnect with nature. It also offers me a greater variety of terrain that is more challenging and more rewarding, and yet kinder to my body. It means freedom! I completed seven off-road ultra marathons in one year, including the 96-mile West Highland Way race. I log many hours on the trails. Some leave me wondering why I put myself through it, but ultimately, they are all so rewarding."

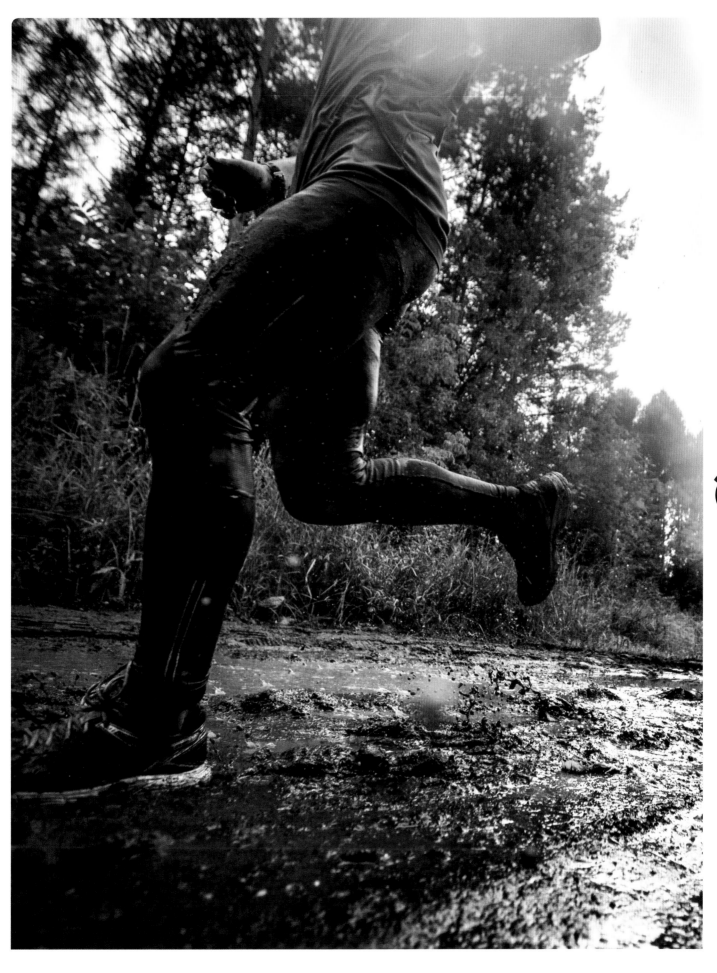

20 OF THE BEST MARATHONS IN THE WORLD

When it comes to marathon running, the world really is your oyster.

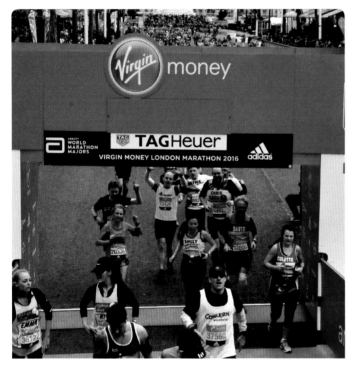

VIRGIN LONDON MARATHON, UK

This fantastic race gets more popular – more than 250,000 people applied for a ballot place in 2017, with almost 40,000 taking part. It features the UK capital's most iconic buildings (including Big Ben and Buckingham Palace), impeccable organisation, a mix of elite and unfeasibly attired fancy-dress runners (think giraffe outfits with 3.6-metre necks) and madly enthusiastic crowds.

DATE – April
www.virginlondonmarathon.com

BIG SUR INTERNATIONAL MARATHON, CALIFORNIA, USA

If you've ever driven from San Francisco to Los Angeles, watching the crashing surf of the Pacific Ocean from the cliff-top road, you'll know why the Big Sur gets such rave reviews. The challenging course starts in Big Sur, follows Highway One – the USA's first nationally designated "scenic highway" – and ends in Carmel-by-the-Sea, where Hollywood legend Clint Eastwood once held office as mayor. The race starts at 6.45 am and buses begin leaving for the start at 3.45am.

DATE – April
www.bsim.org

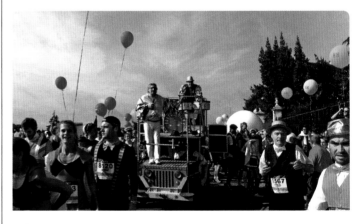

MÉDOC MARATHON, BORDEAUX, FRANCE

Affectionately dubbed the world's longest marathon, because of the extra distance you're likely to cover if you visit every one of this race's 20-something wine-tasting stops. Likened to a carnival procession, fancy dress is pretty much compulsory with a different theme each year. The route wends its way past many of the region's most famous chateaux and also offers opportunities to sample local delicacies, such as oysters, cheese and ham.

DATE – September
www.marathondumedoc.com

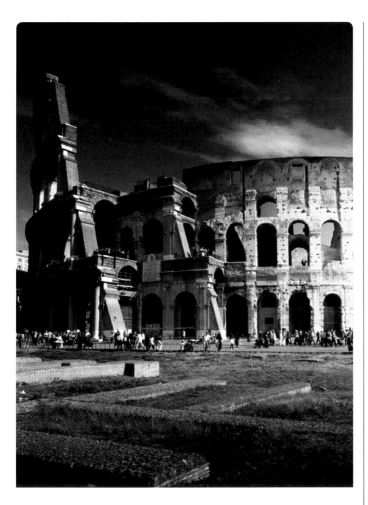

ROME MARATHON, ITALY

Rome is a city built on seven hills, but when you run this race there seem to be many more, which is why so few PBs are set (ankle-endangering cobbled sections don't help). The highly photogenic route starts and finishes near the Colosseum and passes world-famous sights such as the Piazza Navona, the Trevi Fountain and the Spanish Steps.
DATE – March
www.maratonadiroma.it

SOWETO MARATHON, NEAR JOHANNESBURG, SOUTH AFRICA

It's the cheering spectators that make this marathon so special. Starting and finishing at the Elkah stadium, the route takes in many top landmarks, such as Vilakazi Street, which features homes that belonged to Nelson Mandela and Archbishop Desmond Tutu.
DATE – November
www.sowetomarathon.com

PRAGUE INTERNATIONAL MARATHON, CZECH REPUBLIC

Parts of the course are within the historic city, but the flat route also includes sections along the Vltava River. The Czech Republic is renowned for its beer, so don't forget to enjoy an ice-cold Budvar at one of the city's pavement cafés afterwards.
DATE – May
www.praguemarathon.com

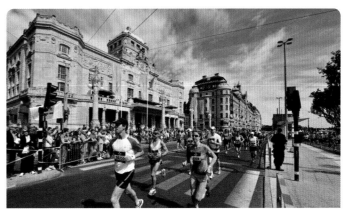

STOCKHOLM MARATHON, SWEDEN

The route of this race passes many of the Swedish capital's most famous buildings and waterways, and crosses the country's largest arched bridge – Västerbron – twice! The stunning setting, carnival atmosphere (complete with showgirl cheerleaders) and finish in the 1912 Olympic Stadium will soon take your mind off the late start – 2.00 pm – and subsequent afternoon heat.
DATE – June
www.stockholmmarathon.se

MIDNIGHT SUN MARATHON, TROMSØ, NORWAY

If you'd like to try running in broad daylight in the middle of the night, this race is held in a city 250 miles north of the Arctic Circle. In midsummer the sun doesn't set for two whole months. Only about 300 runners take on the challenge, which begins at 10.30 pm, but those who do are guaranteed a unique experience.
DATE - June
www.msm.no

BOSTON MARATHON, MASSACHUSETTS, USA

First held in 1897, Boston is the oldest continuously run marathon in the world and one of the toughest races to get into because of its qualifying times. Women aged 18 to 34, for example, have to be able to run a marathon in under 3 hours 35 minutes and even those women over 80 are expected to have completed a 5-hour 25-minute marathon!
DATE – April
www.bostonmarathon.org

BMW BERLIN MARATHON, GERMANY

Few marathons have a more spectacular finish than this one. Running through the Brandenburg Gate, knowing that for many years it formed the boundary between East and West Germany and that you'd risk being shot if you tried to do this during the Cold War, is a thrilling experience. The course is regarded as the fastest in the world – with six records in a row set here between 2003 and 2014, the most recent being Dennis Kimetto (Kenya) with 2 hours 2 minutes 57 seconds.
DATE – September
www.bmw-berlin-marathon.com

BANK OF AMERICA CHICAGO MARATHON, ILLINOIS, USA

Towering skyscrapers, loud and proud crowds, a lakeside setting, a huge field of 45,000 runners and a one-loop fast and flat course are the reasons why many runners rate Chicago as America's best marathon. The route takes you on a tour through many of the lively neighbourhoods that are a world away from the tourist trails.

DATE – October

www.chicagomarathon.com

ZERMATT MARATHON, SWITZERLAND

This energy-sapping race starts in St Niklaus, the lowest-lying mountain valley in Switzerland and then ascends a staggering 1,944 metres, passing the chic ski resort of Zermatt, with views of the Matterhorn and ending at the highest altitude finish line in Europe, the alpine town of Riffelberg. The panoramic views of the Alps will hopefully take your mind off your screaming muscles.

DATE – July

www.zermattmarathon.ch

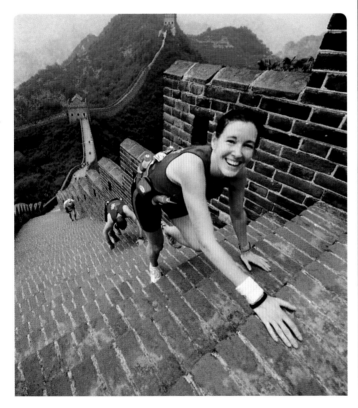

THE GREAT WALL MARATHON, CHINA

Here's where you can hit the wall on the Wall! It takes place in China's Tianjin Province and includes a 7K stretch of the Great Wall itself. Tough but spectacular, the course includes 5,164 steps, as well as asphalt and gravel roads that pass through rural villages and rice fields. The high temperatures and challenges can easily add more than an hour to your standard time on this gruelling-but-gorgeous course.

DATE – May

www.great-wall-marathon.com

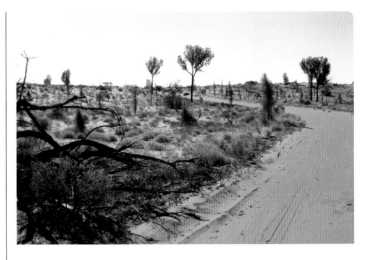

AUSTRALIAN OUTBACK MARATHON

Featuring Uluru (Ayers Rock) as its backdrop, this predominantly off-road two-lap marathon features a mix of relatively flat bush trails, tracks, and sealed and unsealed roads. The average temperature here in July is a running-friendly 21°C.

DATE – July

www.australianoutbackmarathon.com

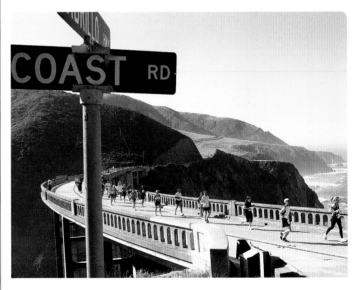

KAISER PERMANENTE NAPA VALLEY MARATHON, CALIFORNIA, USA

A small rural race, that takes you through the lush vineyards near San Francisco. Due to limited course access, crowd support is sparse, but the race's expo, which draws big-name speakers, makes this a world-class event.

DATE – March

www.napavalleymarathon.org

FLORENCE MARATHON, ITALY

Carb-loading the night before at a *trattoria* is just one of the race's many highlights. Set in one of the most architecturally rich cities in the world, it starts in the Piazzale Michelangelo, which boasts spectacular views. After the first 3K, which are a gentle downhill, it wends

its way through some of Florence's most famous squares, following a course that's almost entirely flat.
DATE – November
www.firenzemarathon.it

ABN AMRO MARATHON ROTTERDAM, THE NETHERLANDS

This race offers the second-fastest marathon course in the world and is the Netherlands' biggest one-day sporting event. The only hills you face as you run through Europe's largest port city are the inclines on the bridges and underpasses. Tugboats spray huge arcs of water to welcome you as you cross the Erasmus Bridge, and the route is lined with supporters and live music all the way to the finish.
DATE – April
www.marathonrotterdam.org

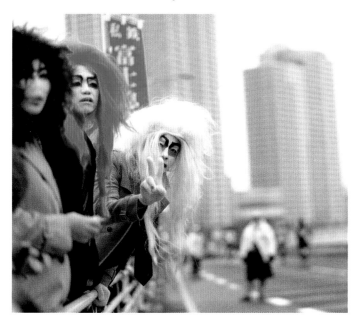

TOKYO MARATHON, JAPAN

One of the youngest international city marathons this race even has a ballot for those who wish to be roadside volunteers and marshals. Starting outside Shinjuku's Metropolitan Government building, the relatively flat route passes the Imperial Palace and traverses downtown Tokyo, cheered on by a million spectators.
DATE – February
www.tokyo42195.org

SEVILLE MARATHON, SPAIN

This well-organised marathon somehow manages to miss virtually all of Seville's attractions and takes you through the city's orange tree-lined streets. Very flat, it's great if you're looking for a PB. The after-race party is included in the price or you can spend the evening medicating your aching limbs with a glass of sangria in one of Seville's tiny tiled tapas bars.
DATE – February
imd.sevilla.org/maraton

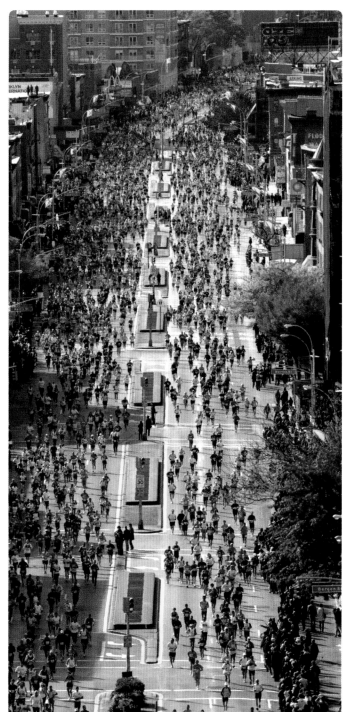

TCS NEW YORK CITY MARATHON, USA

Americans are the world's least-inhibited supporters and you're carried along the streets of New York's five boroughs on a tide of deafening encouragement. One minute you're dwarfed by cloud-shrouded skyscrapers, the next you're tackling one of the five bridges, which provide surprisingly challenging climbs. By the time you reach the finish in Central Park, like the city that's so good they named it twice, you'll want to do it all over again.
DATE – November
www.tcsnycmarathon.org

MOUNTAIN MARATHONS

Cresting a summit is not just the preserve of the hardcore competitor. It can be a realistic goal.

You might think of super-skinny runners disappearing over the hill carrying even super-skinnier rucksacks containing the latest hyper-lightweight mountain tent. But mountain running is more accessible than you realise once you've mastered the basics.

In the UK, for example, events follow the same international format in that the exact location is not announced until a couple of days beforehand to prevent competitors from checking out the area. Races are run in pairs and take place over two days with different categories for different abilities. The elite can expect to cover up to 80 km and be on the go for over 12 hours during the weekend, while lower down the field, runners cover half that distance. They still expect it to take more than eight hours over the two days.

SELF-SUFFICIENCY
Competitors are given a map and a number of grid references that need to be visited in order. The team pairs carry their tent, sleeping bag, stove, food and first aid kit and choose their own route to each of the checkpoints, ending with an overnight camp. The process is repeated the following day.

While there is no pounding a hard surface at a steady pace, competitors need to be able to keep going over rough ground for a long time. The ability to put up with discomfort is the key. Both partners need to run carrying a rucksack and then share a tiny damp tent with a sweaty partner. There is a distinct lack of hot showers and gourmet food but the camaraderie at the overnight camp and on the hill makes up for the hardship.

THE BASICS
The ability to navigate is essential. The routes cover rough, open ground rather than paths and a sound knowledge of using a map and compass is required. Smartphones are not allowed and neither are GPS devices. Competitors will need to have some experience being in hill environments, but navigating is a more important skill than being able to run fast. Taking time to study the map and choosing the best route is vital.

The elite runners keep up the pace; in reality most of the competitors in the easier categories will walk up the hills taking in the beauty of their surroundings. A slower pace

also gives participants a chance to double-check the map and avoid making hasty route choices. The checkpoints are located so they can be reached without entering dangerous terrain and rock-climbing skills are not needed, although confidence on steep ground is expected.

MOUNTAIN TRAINING
You should be familiar with the basic endurance training that you would do for a long road race, but remember that in a mountain marathon you will be on the go for many hours. Forget what you know about mile paces and be prepared to go slower for longer. You will need to find hilly training routes, ideally in the countryside, for your long runs and get used to running with a rucksack. You can also find organisations that help with training on the specifics of navigation and running.

MOUNTAIN EQUIPMENT

Some people will tell tales of competitors cutting off their excess shoelaces to save weight but first timers need not go to such extremes. You will see elite pairs with their micro-loads but there will also be folk with their standard rucksacks so you needn't be intimidated. In addition to any emergency kit required by the organiser you will need:
• Trail or fell shoes are essential for grip on wet grass and loose rock
• Waterproof jacket and bottoms
• Tent – some competitors may squeeze into a tiny tent but others value comfort over weight and opt for a two-man
• Lightweight sleeping bag – which will probably take up most space in your pack
• Sleeping mat
• Stove and fuel
• Mug and pot
• Rucksack – remember, you are in a pair so you can share the load

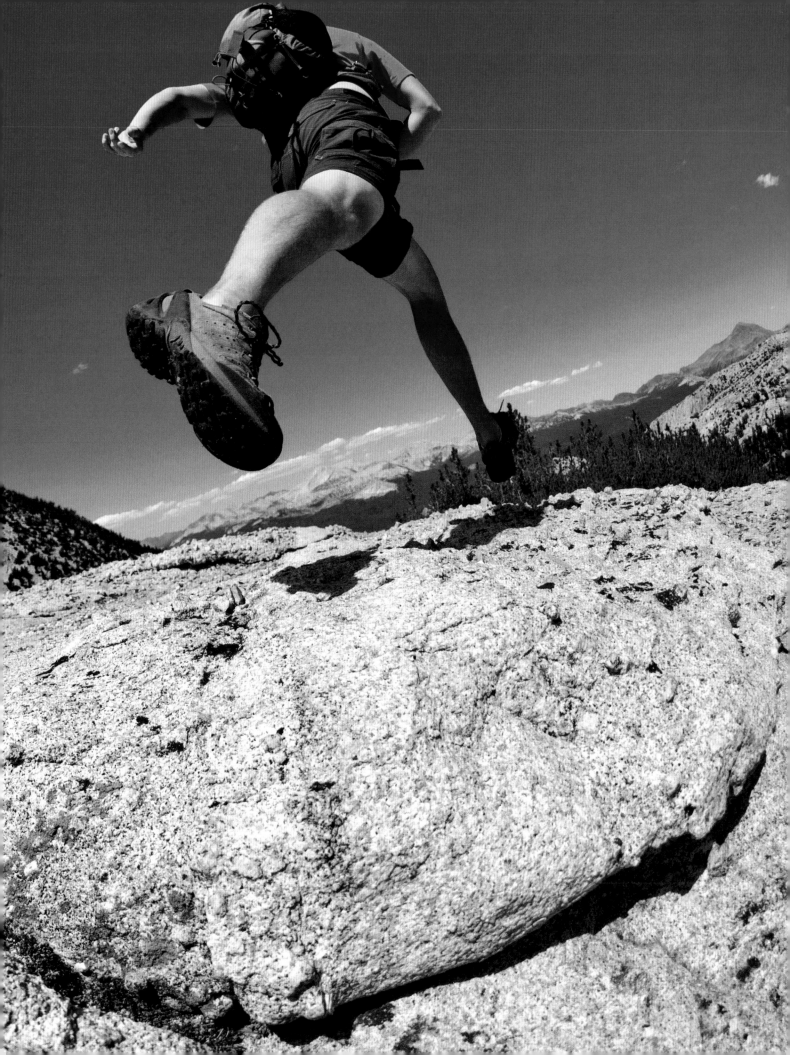

FELL RUNNING

The scenery in fell running - also known as hill running - will take your breath away, but it can be tough.

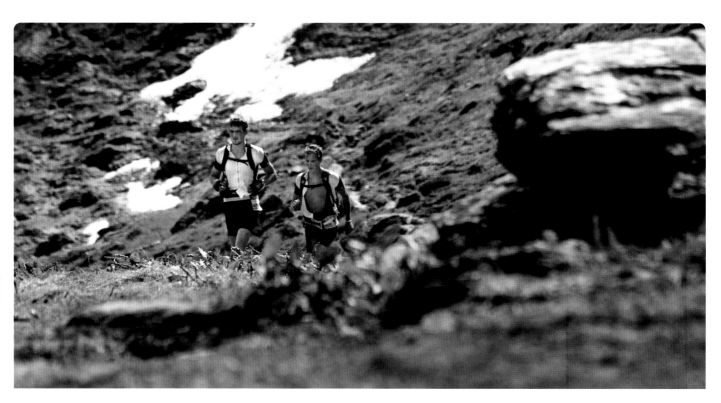

Take a trail run and add steeper slopes, rock, scree, extreme weather conditions and heart-stopping views, and you have a fell run. Usually associated with hardcore athleticism, fell running isn't as inaccessible to mere mortals as it may seem. There are daunting races (such as the UK's Bob Graham Round in the Lake District, which involves scaling 42 summits within 24 hours) and they do push runners to their limits, but there are also shorter, gentler fell runs that are becoming more popular among regular runners.

Of course, the main difference between fell running and everyday trail running is the mountainous terrain. There is nothing as wild and, in turn, as addictive, as leaving your email and your mobile phone in the car and heading up into the misty peaks. In the words of Richard Askwith in his iconic book *Feet in the Clouds*:

"The point is not the exertion involved. It's the degree of involvement, or immersion, in the landscape. You need to feel it, to interact with it; to be in it, not just looking from the outside. You need to lose yourself – for it is then that you are most human."

The wildness and freedom of powering over the high fells, with the responsibilities of modern life no more than a memory somewhere below, make it addictive. But if you fancy giving it a go, there are some adjustments in training, kit and safety precautions to make first.

TRAINING

Fell running is tough on the body, in particular the control muscles (such as the core), which give you the balance and strength to run at pace downhill, and the thigh muscles, which power you up those steep gradients. "When we run uphill, the quadriceps are particularly used, in order to create upward drive," explained physiotherapist Holly King. "The contraction of the four muscles within the thigh needs to be balanced and strong, to produce the power required for propulsion up slopes and to prevent injury." Novice fell runners can strengthen their quadriceps by doing cross training, such as breaststroke, cycling or hill walking and their core muscles by doing Pilates, yoga or dance. There are also specific exercises you can do at home:

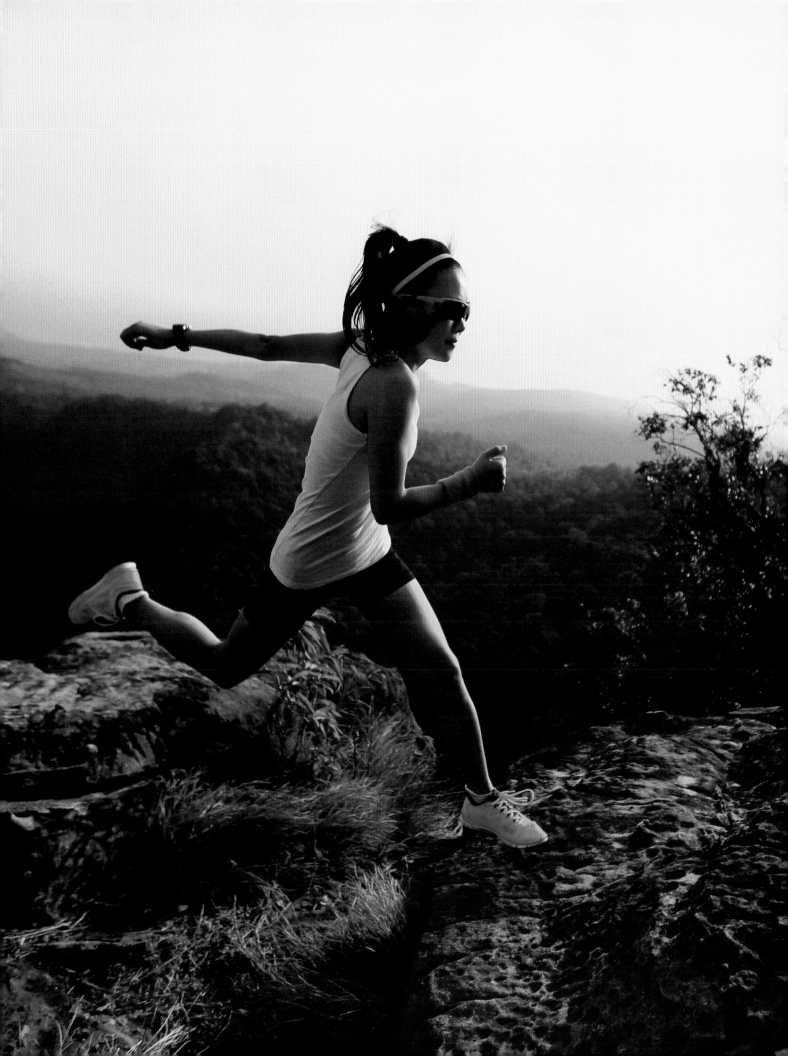

DEEP SQUATS

EFFECT – creates stability in the knee area
AREA TRAINED – glutes
TECHNIQUE
• Tie a resistance band above your knees.
• Stand with your feet slightly wider than hip-width apart and turn your feet out. Then squat.
• Over time, increase the depth of the bend and the amount of squats you do.

LEG STEPS

EFFECT – develops leg control to run down steep hills
AREA TRAINED – quadriceps
TECHNIQUE
• Stand on a step, lower your opposite leg and bend your knee with control.
• Your knee should stay above your toes.
• Gradually increase the amount of leg steps you do over time.

BALANCING

EFFECT – Stability to run uphill
AREA TRAINED – core
TECHNIQUE
• Stand on one leg and take the other leg up in front of your chest.
• Stretch the leg back behind you, ensuring your pelvis remains level.
• Bring it back to the starting point and change sides.

THE ONLY WAY ISN'T UP

As with mountain running (see pp.162–163), as well as taking the right kit with you, it's vital to know how to use it. If you're not a proficient map reader, ask somebody who is to teach you. Eric Langmuir's book *Mountaincraft and Leadership* has lots of tips for mastering navigation on the fells. It's important to be responsible for your own navigation. Most fell races don't have marked courses, so you must find your own path and the runner in front won't necessarily be going the right way. Take note of the landmarks you are passing (trees and boulders, etc.) in case you have to retrace your steps.

When starting out, it's a good idea to hook up with some experienced fell runners for safety, camaraderie and tips. Start out on some of the lower fells before tackling the big peaks and run when weather conditions are kind. If you want to really get into the sport, it's worth joining a club.

Last but not least, start out slowly. Your times on roads and regular trails will not translate onto the fells and if you start off like the clappers, you'll exhaust yourself. Pace the route gradually, so you leave enough in the tank to get back down the hill.

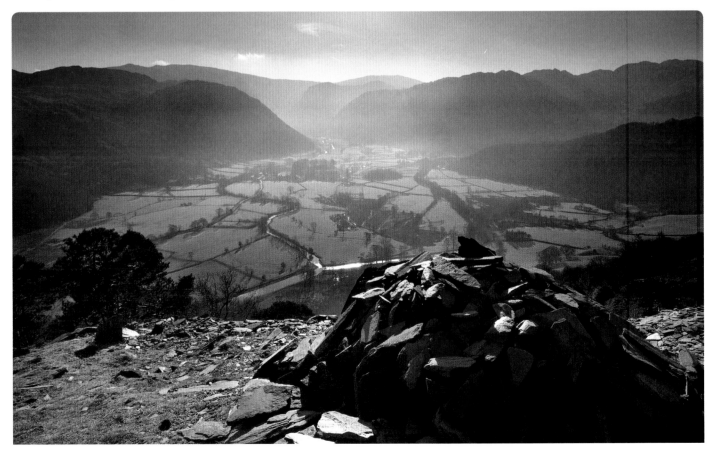

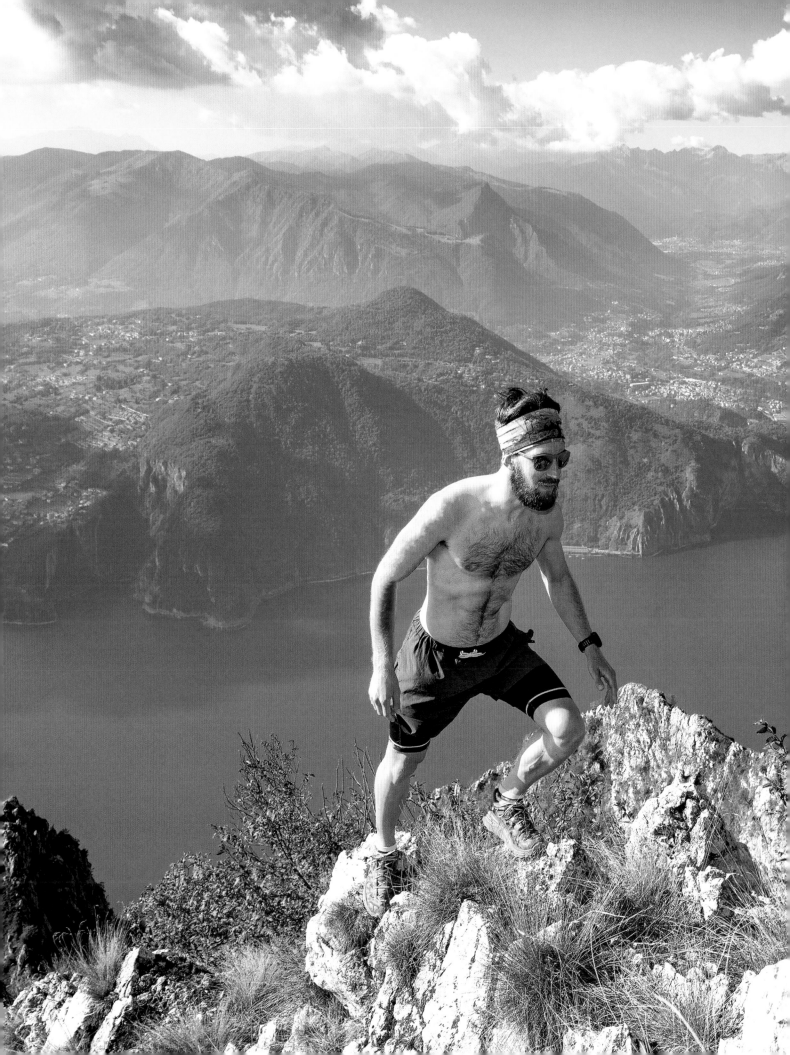

EFFICIENT BREATHING

It's the most natural thing in the world, but many runners breathe incorrectly.

Most of us only use about two-thirds of our available lung space at the best of times, and the rest of us take small, shallow sips of air, increasing the tension in our already overloaded systems. Watch a baby breathe and you will see its stomach lift and lower as the air enters and leaves the body. This is how we were designed to breathe. Watch a typical adult when they breathe: the chest may move but the abdomen is probably going to stay still and this shows that we are not using our diaphragms properly.

"Running requires aerobic respiration," said sports physician Dr Geoff Davies, "which means it needs higher breathing rates for more oxygen and higher heart rates to supply this oxygen to your exercising muscles."

BREATHING FOR BEGINNERS

168

Although breathing is supposed to be instinctive, many new runners struggle and even give up because they feel they can't control their breath. However, the more you practise, the easier it will become. "The important thing is to concentrate on taking full, deep, regular and relaxed breaths rather than quick, shallow breaths,' said Dr Stuart Packham, consultant general physician in respiratory medicine. "This is a more economical way of breathing and is helped by maintaining the correct body posture, particularly of the chest and head."

Always warm up with a fast walk then slow jog before you begin running. This gives your body a chance to prepare for the challenge ahead, and your heart rate and breathing will slowly increase as your body adapts.

BREATHE TO THE RHYTHM

Music can be a very powerful influence on your rhythm – listen to different songs and choose a selection with a similar cadence to your foot fall when running, and then focus on the beat of the music. Tension can increase your heart rate and breathing and tighten your muscles, making your run a struggle. If you are tense, or beginning to struggle, slow down, take a couple of deep breaths in through the nose and out through the mouth.

Practise cadence breathing – elite runners will usually be running at around two foot strikes per inhale and two per exhale, or at a very fast pace, 2:1 (two steps inhale, one exhale). You could start off with a 3:3 cadence and play with the ratio until you find the right numbers to suit your pace

and fitness (be careful not to go too fast too soon, such as 2:2 or 2:1, as you could become light-headed).

YOGIC BREATHING

When you are doing more intensive work such as interval training, your breathing will be much more forced and you will be using different muscles to help get maximum oxygen flow. You can practise full yogic breathing to train your respiratory muscles. Lie on the floor and slowly inhale through your nose for a count of six to eight. Feel the air fill your abdomen, then your chest and then finally feel your collar bones lift as you fully expand your chest. Slowly exhale, feeling each part sink back down and continue exhaling until your abdomen is flattened out and empty for a count of six to eight.

ASTHMA AND HAY FEVER

If you struggle with your breath you can find this causes anxiety. Dr Packham said, "If runners are using their reliever therapy more than twice a week, then their underlying asthma may require additional treatment and it's important that they seek medical advice."

• Yoga – not only will the exercises help to relax you, but also the breathing exercises can really make a difference.
• Pilates – stretches out your ribs and torso and focuses on controlling and slowing the breath.
• Pollution – try to exercise away from traffic fumes.
• Indoor – in weather extremes you may be better off training at the gym as excess cold or heat can become an irritant.

"If you are tense or beginning to struggle, slow down, and take a couple of deep breaths in through the nose and out through the mouth."

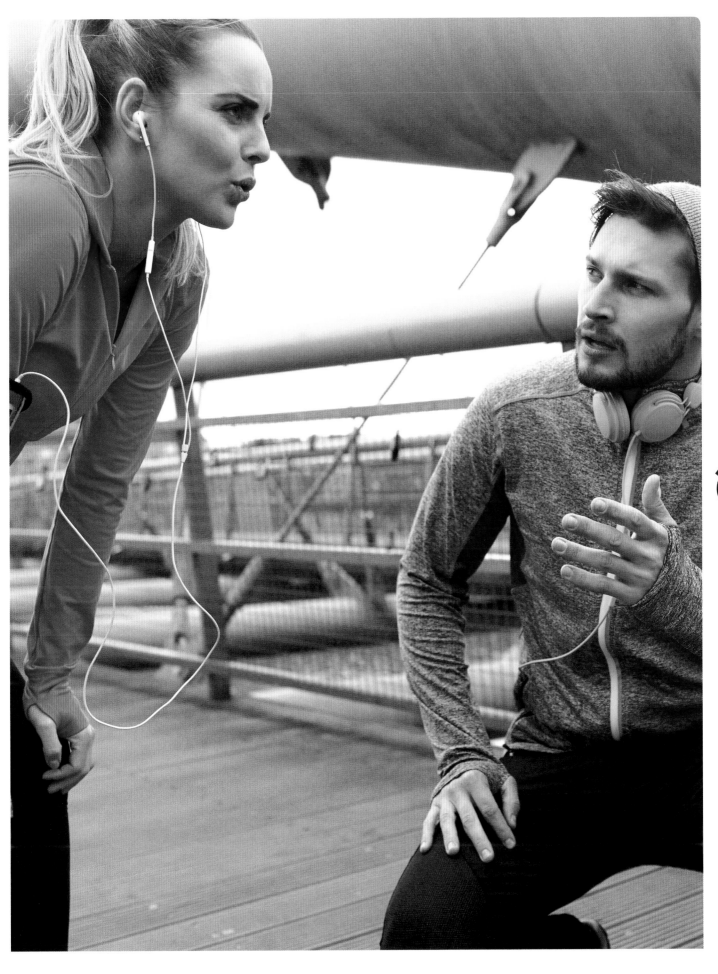

169

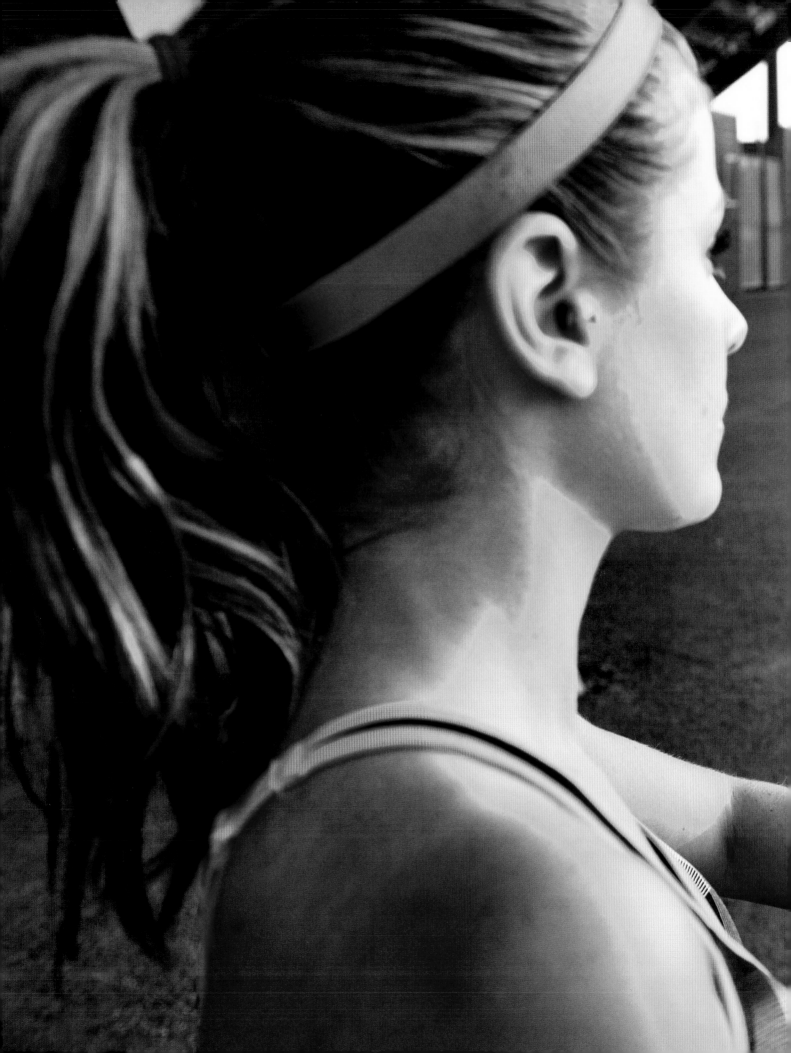

TRAINING PLANS

Here's some programmes for 5K, 10K, half-marathon and marathons. These target both beginners and improvers and feature insider tips and ideas for development for each distance. The week-by-week plans are all you need to complete the race of your choice - good luck with whichever event you choose!

5K TRAINING PLAN FOR BEGINNERS

172

	DAY 1	DAY 2	DAY 3	DAY 4	DAY 5	DAY 6	DAY 7
WEEK 1	Run 1 min / walk 2 mins x 5 = 15 mins	Rest	Run 1 min / walk 1 min x 5 = 10 mins	Rest / stretch	Rest or gentle swim or cycle for 15 mins	Run / walk 15 mins with as few walk breaks as possible	Rest or yoga class
WEEK 2	Run 1 min / walk 2 mins x 6 = 18 mins	Rest	Run 2 mins / walk 1 min x 6 = 18mins	Rest / stretch	Rest or swim or cycle for 20 mins	Run / walk 20 mins with as few walk breaks as possible	Rest or yoga class
WEEK 3	Run 2 mins / walk 2 mins x 6 = 24 mins	Rest	Run 3 mins / walk 1 min x 4 = 16 mins	Rest / stretch	Rest or swim or cycle for 22 mins	Run / walk 25 mins with as few walk breaks as possible	Rest or yoga class
WEEK 4	Run 3 mins / walk 2 mins x 4 = 20 mins	Rest	Run 3 mins / walk 2 mins x 4 = 20 mins	Rest / stretch	Rest or swim or cycle for 25 mins	Run / walk 30 mins with as few walk breaks as possible	Rest or yoga class
WEEK 5	Run 5 mins / walk 2 mins x 3 = 21 mins	Rest	Run 4 mins / walk 1 min x 5 = 25 mins	Rest / stretch	Rest or swim or cycle for 25 mins	Run / walk 35 mins with as few walk breaks as possible	Rest or yoga class
WEEK 6	Run 6 mins / walk 1 min x 4 = 28mins	Rest	Run 5 mins / walk 1 min x 4 = 24 mins	Rest / stretch	Rest or swim or cycle for 30 mins	Run / walk 40 mins with as few walk breaks as possible	Rest or yoga class
WEEK 7	Run 7 mins / walk 1 min x 3 = 24mins	Rest	Run 8 mins / walk 1 min x 3 = 27 mins	Rest / stretch	Rest or swim or cycle for 35 mins	Run / walk 45 mins with as few walk breaks as possible	Rest or yoga class
WEEK 8	Run 8 mins / walk 1 min x 4 = 36mins	Rest	Run 25 mins	Rest / stretch	Rest or swim or cycle for 30 mins	Rest	5K run day – good luck!

5K TRAINING PLAN FOR IMPROVERS

	DAY 1	DAY 2	DAY 3	DAY 4	DAY 5	DAY 6	DAY 7
WEEK 1	Run 20 mins Walk 5 mins Run 5 mins at faster pace	Rest	Run 20 mins Strength training & stretching	Rest	Hill training: 20 mins hill repeats - run up; jog down to recover	Rest	Run 30 mins
WEEK 2	Rest	Run 20 mins Strength training & stretching	Rest	Sprint training: 5 mins warm up 1 min fast running 1 min recovery repeat x 10 5 mins cooldown	Rest	Run 35 mins	Swim or cycle
WEEK 3	Run 20 mins Walk 5 mins Run 10 mins at faster pace	Rest	Run 30 mins Strength training & stretching	Rest	Hill training: 30 mins hill repeats - run up; jog down to recover	Rest	Run 40 mins
WEEK 4	Rest	Run 30 mins Strength training & stretching	Rest	Cross trainer / swim or bike 45 mins	Rest	Rest	Run 40 mins alternating 5 mins easy; 5mins pushing the pace
WEEK 5	Rest	Run 30 mins Strength training & stretching	Rest	Sprint training: 5 mins warm up 1min fast running 1 min recovery repeat x 10 5 mins cool down	Rest	Run 30 mins pushing pace throughout	Rest
WEEK 6	Run 20 mins Strength training & stretching	Rest	Hill training: 30 mins hill repeats - run up; jog down to recover	Easy 20 min run	Rest	Rest	Run 5K

5K IN UNDER 20 MINUTES

How much work you need to put in depends on how close you are to that magical teen-time. The most important thing is not to rush. The moment you start becoming impatient, you become frustrated and everything else suffers. You will also start rushing or pushing yourself more than you should, which will lead to injuries.

Doing three different sessions a week is a must and they should include, in no particular order: an intervals session, a 5-10 mile run and a 5K run.

THE KEY SESSIONS

INTERVALS – here you're building up your speed endurance – your ability to run faster, longer. You should be running around 80–90 per cent of your max speed, so considerably quicker than 5K pace. Try six by two minutes with a minute rest in between each rep. Do one, two, three, three, two and one minutes, with a minute rest between each rep. Or 30, 60, 90, 90, 60 and 30-second reps with a 45-second rest between.

5-10 MILE RUN – whether you can muster 5 or 10 miles, this is still important. Running further than your desired distance will build both stamina and fitness. Hand in hand with your intervals, being able to run longer for faster will make you even quicker over short periods. It's common sense, right?

5K RUNS – practice really does make perfect: getting used to the distance and what your body can achieve is crucial to getting your time down. If you feel like you want to add more training, than resistance work is great. Using your own body weight for press-ups and crunches will improve strength and power. Work your way up through the weeks.

NUTRITION

Being a runner is about lean strength. The lower your body fat the better. Depending on whether you're looking to make the time just once or to keep regularly hitting below the 20-minute mark could be the difference between a temporary or total lifestyle change. Many diets need very little changing; it's usually just a case of cutting out the crisps, chocolate and fast food. After the first couple of weeks, you can reward yourself with a slither of chocolate on a Friday or a glass of wine.

Pacing will be key. Setting off too quickly is a problem for even the best runners. Keeping the same pace is the best way of assuring you have enough left in the tank for a sprint finish. This is why practicing 5K runs becomes even more crucial. Admittedly, this is very hard to do without a device – having a running watch which can guide you is a great way of keeping you on track. Aiming for four minutes each kilometre will mean you're on target for 20. Keep aiming for those four minutes and eventually you'll get down to it. If you can't afford a watch, there are plenty of free apps on your smart phone too. Failing that, a regular stopwatch to count your minutes should work just as fine.

ON THE DAY OF THE RACE

Keep things very simple. If you're running on a weekend for example, just one gentle run on the previous Wednesday will be fine. As with any race, be sure you try nothing new on the day: eat what you've always eaten and drink what you have always drunk. For the two nights leading up to the event, try and get at least seven hours' sleep. You'll be surprised how much this actually helps. There's nothing quite like feeling refreshed on the day. Make sure you have the practicalities ready a day in advance: where you're going, what you're wearing and what you're taking with you. It is so important to have as little stress before the race as possible so that you feel completely ready on the start line

"For the two nights leading up to the event, try and get at least seven hours' sleep."

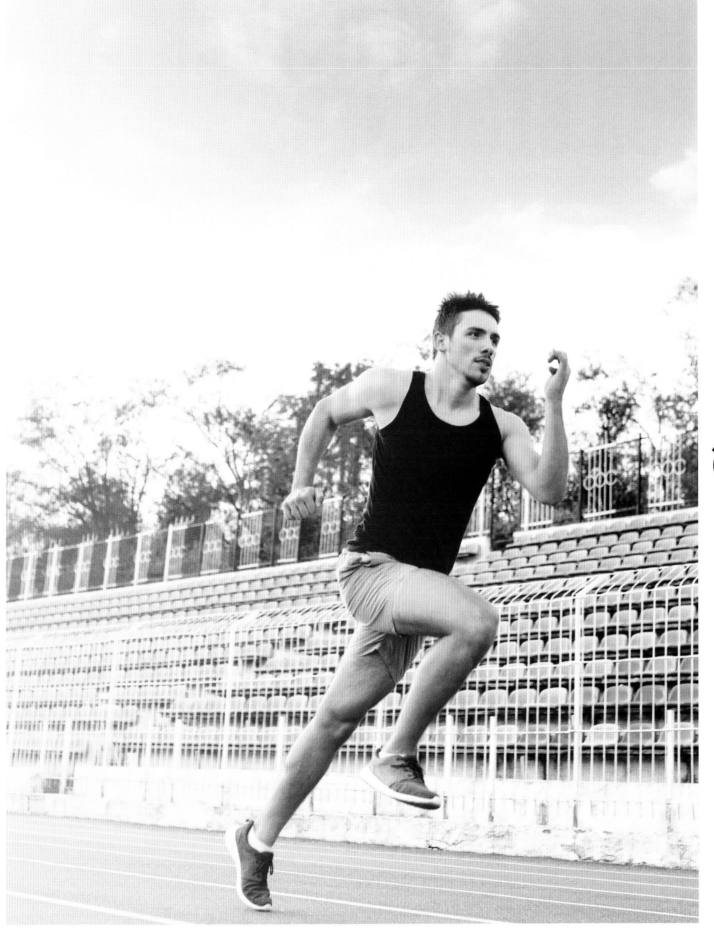

10K TRAINING PLAN FOR BEGINNERS

	DAY 1	DAY 2	DAY 3	DAY 4	DAY 5	DAY 6	DAY 7
WEEK 1	Walk / run 20 mins	Walk / run 20 mins	Rest	Walk / run 30 mins	Rest	Run 10 mins Strength training & stretching	Walk / run 30 mins
WEEK 2	Rest	Walk / run 25 mins Run 5 mins	Rest	Run 10 mins Walk 5 mins Run 10 mins	Strength training & stretching	Rest	Walk / run 40 mins
WEEK 3	Rest	Run 12 mins Walk 5 mins Run 12 mins	Cross training / circuit class / swim / bike for 45 mins	Run 15 mins Strength training & stretching	Rest	Run 15 mins Walk 5 mins Run 10 mins Walk 3 mins Run 5 mins	Run 20 mins
WEEK 4	Rest	Run 20 mins Walk 5 mins Run 15 mins	Rest	Run 20 mins Strength training & stretching	Rest	Rest	Run 5 mins easy 2 mins faster repeat x 6
WEEK 5	Rest	Hill training 25 mins hill repeats - run up; jog down to recover	Rest	Run 20 mins Strength training & stretching	Cross training / circuit class / swim / bike for 45 mins	Rest	Run 30 mins Run 5 mins faster Run 15 mins
WEEK 6	Rest	Hill training 25 mins hill repeats - run up; jog down to recover	Run 20 mins Strength training & stretching	Rest	Run 20-30 mins easy	Rest	Run 10k

10K TRAINING PLAN FOR IMPROVERS

	DAY 1	DAY 2	DAY 3	DAY 4	DAY 5	DAY 6	DAY 7
WEEK 1	Run 30 mins	Rest	Run 20 mins Strength training & stretching	Rest	Hill training: 30 mins hill repeats - run up; jog down to recover	Rest	Run 45 mins
WEEK 2	Rest	Run 5 mins warm up 5 mins quick 5 mins easy repeat x3	Rest	Run 20 mins Strength training & stretching	Cross training / circuit class / swim / bike for 45 mins	Rest	Run 45 mins
WEEK 3	Run 30 mins Run 5 mins fast	Rest	Run 20 mins Strength training & stretching	Rest	Rest	Hill training: 30 mins hill repeats - run up; jog down to recover	Run 45 mins
WEEK 4	Rest	Run 20 mins Strength training & stretching	Rest	Run 30 mins Run 5 mins fast Run 10 mins	Cross training / circuit class / swim / bike for 45 mins	Rest	Run 5 mins easy Run 5 mins fast Repeat x 5
WEEK 5	Run 20 mins	Rest	Run 30 mins Strength training & stretching	Run 40 mins	Rest	Rest	Run 5 mins easy Run 5 mins fast Repeat x 6
WEEK 6	Rest	Run 30 mins Strength training & stretching	Cross training / circuit class / swim / bike for 45 mins	Rest	Run 20 mins easy	Rest	Run 10k

10 WEEKS TO A 10K PB

10K races require a tricky combo of speed and endurance. You can put together a ten-week programme of sessions to make it happen.

The 10K is a challenging distance at speed. The pace and effort will mean you're closer to your VO2 max for most of the race. Build your fitness and learn to defeat the fatigue, oxygen debt and gremlins in the mind telling you to stop. The 10–12 week training period leading up to your 10K should weekly include a long run, a threshold session and one of the sessions below. You might add some morning easy runs, a fartlek or wind-up run. Keep core conditioning and cross-training in the schedule. These progressive sessions start ten weeks before race day and peak in the penultimate week of training, allowing the final session to be part of your pre-race taper.

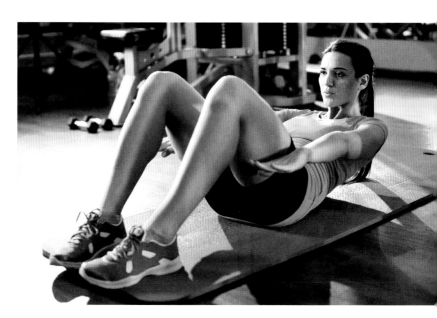

TEN SESSIONS: ONE A WEEK

1 6 X 5-MINUTE INTERVALS ON THE ROAD OR TRACK WITH 75-90 SECONDS JOG RECOVERY

Run numbers 1–3 at threshold effort and 4–6 at your target 10K pace. Aim to run the second half of this session quicker than the first.

2 8-10 X 800 M OR 3-MINUTE INTERVALS WITH 5-90 SECONDS RECOVERY

Run the odd numbers (1, 3, 5, 7, 9) at threshold effort and the even numbers at target 10K pace.

Another larger volume session that makes you think about pace and effort.

Alternating with threshold allows you to complete the full workout.

3 4-5 X 1 MILE OR 6 MINUTES AT TARGET 10K PACE WITH A 90-SECOND JOG RECOVERY

This always hurts but is a classic 10K session.

4 THE LONG FARTLEK

Aim to run for 60 minutes but include blocks of 6 minutes, 5 minutes, 4 minutes, 3 minutes, 2 minutes, 1 minute, all with a 90-second jog/run recovery.

Each block should be a fraction quicker than the last. Run the first block at threshold pace.

5 10 MINUTES AT THRESHOLD (3 MINUTES RECOVERY) PLUS 5-6 X 800 M WITH NUMBERS 1-3 AT 10K PACE AND 4-6 AT 5K PACE ALL WITH 90 SECONDS RECOVERY (3 MINUTES RECOVERY) + 10 MINUTES AT THRESHOLD PACE

A clever session with big volumes of running but different paces for building endurance.

There will be tough moments during these sessions.

6 8-10 X 1K OR 3.5 MINUTES ALL AT TARGET 10K PACE WITH 75-90 SECONDS RECOVERY

This is another classic session – don't run faster than your target 10K time. Finish strongly and pick up the pace with the final few reps.

7 RUN A 5K PARKRUN OR GPS TIME TRIAL AT YOUR TARGET 10K PACE. TAKE A 5-10 MINUTE JOG RECOVERY THEN COMPLETE 5 X 2 MINUTES AT YOUR 5K PACE WITH A 2-MINUTE JOG RECOVERY

This is a test of mental strength, working hard.

8 THE WIND-UP SESSION

Run 2K or 6–7 minutes at threshold (2–3 minutes jog recovery).

Complete 4 x 1K at 10K pace with 75–90 seconds jog recovery.

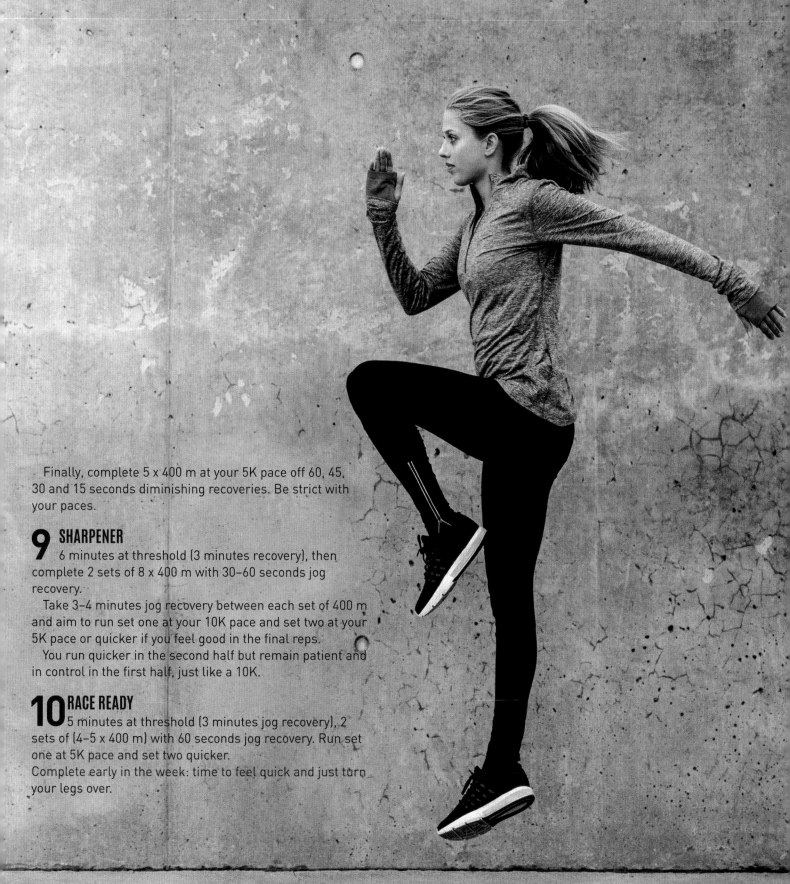

Finally, complete 5 x 400 m at your 5K pace off 60, 45, 30 and 15 seconds diminishing recoveries. Be strict with your paces.

9 SHARPENER

6 minutes at threshold (3 minutes recovery), then complete 2 sets of 8 x 400 m with 30–60 seconds jog recovery.

Take 3–4 minutes jog recovery between each set of 400 m and aim to run set one at your 10K pace and set two at your 5K pace or quicker if you feel good in the final reps.

You run quicker in the second half but remain patient and in control in the first half, just like a 10K.

10 RACE READY

5 minutes at threshold (3 minutes jog recovery), 2 sets of (4–5 x 400 m) with 60 seconds jog recovery. Run set one at 5K pace and set two quicker.

Complete early in the week: time to feel quick and just turn your legs over.

HALF-MARATHON TRAINING PLAN FOR BEGINNERS

	DAY 1	DAY 2	DAY 3	DAY 4	DAY 5	DAY 6	DAY 7
WEEK 1	Run / walk 15 mins	Rest	Run / walk 20 mins	Strength training & stretching	Rest	Run / walk 30 mins	Rest
WEEK 2	Run / walk 20 mins Strength training & stretching	Rest	Run 10 mins Walk 5 mins Run 5 mins	Cross training / circuit class / swim / bike 45 mins	Rest	Run 10 mins Walk 5 mins Repeat x 3	Rest
WEEK 3	Run 5 mins Walk 5 mins Repeat x 4	Rest	Run 10 mins Walk 5 mins Repeat x 3	Rest	Run 15 mins Strength training & stretching	Rest	Run / walk 40 mins
WEEK 4	Cross training / circuit class / swim / bike 45 mins	Run 20 mins Walk 5 mins Run 10 mins	Rest	Run 20 mins Strength training & stretching	Rest	Run 20 mins Walk 5 mins Run 15 mins	Run / walk 50 mins
WEEK 5	Rest	Run 20 mins Walk 5 mins Run 10 mins Walk 5 mins Run 10 mins	Rest	Run 20 mins Strength training & stretching	Rest	Rest	Run / walk 60 mins with as few breaks as possible
WEEK 6	Rest	Run 20 mins Walk 5 mins Run 15 mins	Rest	Run 20 mins Strength training & stretching	Cross training / circuit class / swim / bike 45 mins	Rest	Run 25 mins Walk 5 mins Run 15 mins
WEEK 7	Rest	Run 30 mins Strength training & stretching	Rest	Run 15 mins Strength training & stretching	Run 30 mins	Rest	Run / walk 60 mins with as few breaks as possible
WEEK 8	Cross training / circuit class / swim / bike 45 mins	Rest	Run 45 mins	Rest	Run 20 mins Strength training & stretching	Rest	Run / walk 75 mins with as few breaks as possible
WEEK 9	Run 20 mins	Rest	Run 50 mins	Rest	Run 20 mins Strength training & stretching	Rest	Run 75 mins
WEEK 10	Cross training / circuit class / swim / bike 45 mins	Rest	Run 30 mins Walk 5 mins Run 30 mins	Rest	Run 20 mins Strength training & stretching	Rest	Run 90 mins
WEEK 11	Rest	Run 30 mins	Rest	Run 20 mins Strength training & stretching	Run 30 mins	Rest	Run 105 mins
WEEK 12	Rest	Run 20 mins Strength training & stretching	Rest	Swim	Run 30 mins easy	Rest	Run Half Marathon

HALF-MARATHON TRAINING PLAN FOR IMPROVERS

	DAY 1	DAY 2	DAY 3	DAY 4	DAY 5	DAY 6	DAY 7
WEEK 1	Run 30 mins	Rest	Hill training 30 mins	Rest	Strength training & stretching	Rest	Run 45 mins
WEEK 2	Rest	Run 30 mins Fast run for 5 mins Run 15mins	Rest	Run 30 mins Strength training & stretching	Cross training / circuit class / swim / bike 45 mins	Rest	Run 50 mins incl. 5 mins easy 5 mins faster x 5
WEEK 3	Run 30 mins	Rest	Run 30 mins Strength training & stretching	Rest	Hill training 40 mins	Rest	Run 60 mins
WEEK 4	Cross training / circuit class / swim / bike 45 mins	Rest	Sprint training 5 min warm up 200m sprint 2 mins recovery Repeat x 6	Rest	Run 30 mins Strength training & stretching	Rest	Run 60 mins incl. 5 mins easy 5 mins faster x 6
WEEK 5	Rest	Run 30 mins Strength training & stretching	Rest	Hill training 45 mins	Rest	Rest	Run 60 mins incl. 5 mins easy 10 mins faster x 4
WEEK 6	Rest	Run 30 mins Strength training & stretching	Rest	Sprint training 5 min warm up 400m sprint 4 mins recovery Repeat x 4	Cross training / circuit class / swim / bike 45 mins	Rest	Run 75 mins
WEEK 7	Rest	Run 45 mins	Rest	Run 30 mins Strength training & stretching	Rest	Rest	Run 75 mins incl. 5 mins easy 10 mins faster x 5
WEEK 8	Rest	Run 30 mins Strength training & stretching	Rest	Hill training 45 mins	Cross training / circuit class / swim / bike 45 mins	Rest	Run 90 mins
WEEK 9	Rest	Run 30 mins Strength training & stretching	Rest	Sprint training 5 min warm up 800m sprint 5 mins recovery Repeat x 3	Rest	Rest	Run 90 mins incl. 5 mins easy 5 mins faster x 9
WEEK 10	Rest	Run 30 mins Strength training & stretching	Rest	Hill training 45 mins	Rest	Rest	Run 100 mins
WEEK 11	Rest	Sprint training 5 min warm up 400m sprint 4 mins recovery Repeat x 4	Rest	Hill training 45 mins	Rest	Rest	Run 110 mins
WEEK 12	Rest	Run 30 mins Strength training & stretching	Rest	Easy 30 min run	Swim	Rest	Run Half Marathon

181

13.1 TIPS FOR YOUR FIRST HALF MARATHON

Keep note of these handy facts from threshold running to post-run refreshment.

1 MILES 9-11 ARE MAKE-OR-BREAK
The half marathon may not have a wall, but there's no doubting that miles 9–11 are where PB dreams are made or broken. Dig deep, suffer now and celebrate afterwards.

2 THE HALF DOESN'T REQUIRE HIGH-MILEAGE TRAINING
Unlike the marathon, where you need to focus more on mileage, you can comfortably train for a half marathon on just three runs a week.

3 BUT YOU CAN'T BLAG IT
Thirteen-point-one miles is a long way. Don't try to wing it on the day; respect the distance and put in the training.

4 GO EASY ON THE GELS
If you're going to be finished inside two hours, you can get by with one or two gels. In fact, you will come across some runners who carry no gels at all.

5 DON'T TRAIN TOO FAST
If your training consists solely of quick 5Ks, you may find that you struggle in the latter half of the race. Make sure you include a weekly long run where the focus is on distance rather than speed.

6 DON'T TRAIN TOO SLOW
If your training consists solely of one-pace plodding, you're unlikely to finish in a quick time. The half-marathon requires both speed and endurance so make sure you do some sharper runs mid-week.

7 THE BEGINNER OPTION
While the idea of running 26.2 miles is pretty daunting, the half-marathon is a little friendlier. That said, if it is your first half marathon, enter a 10K race as part of your training.

8 TRY TEMPO RUNNING
You will run at about 75 per cent of your maximum effort. It's absolutely ideal for the half as it will help boost both your speed and endurance. Aim for ten minutes of tempo work to start with, and build it up from there.

9 FIND YOUR THRESHOLD
Testing – both physically and mentally – but nailing them will hugely help you in your half marathon.

10 KNOW THE COURSE
Is it flat and fast, or hilly and challenging? Knowing the course will help to prepare you for what lies ahead. There's nothing worse than heading to a race hoping for a PB only to find there's a huge hill about four miles in. Do your research and pick your race accordingly.

11 BEWARE: THE HALF MARATHON MAY LEAD YOU ON
Once the pain in your legs has subsided, your thoughts may well turn to the marathon distance.

12 THE IDEAL DISTANCE
Some people choose to specialise at the half marathon distance. Requiring less training and taking less of a toll on your body than the marathon, you can run them fairly regularly and keep snipping away at your PB.

13 BRING SUPPORTERS
Knowing there will be a few friendly faces in the crowd can be a real boost on race-day. Position your posse where they'll be most needed – probably around the ten-mile mark – and let their goodwill propel you to the finish.

13.1 CELEBRATE
No half marathon is complete without a little post-run celebration. Arrange to meet a few of your supporters and toast your success.

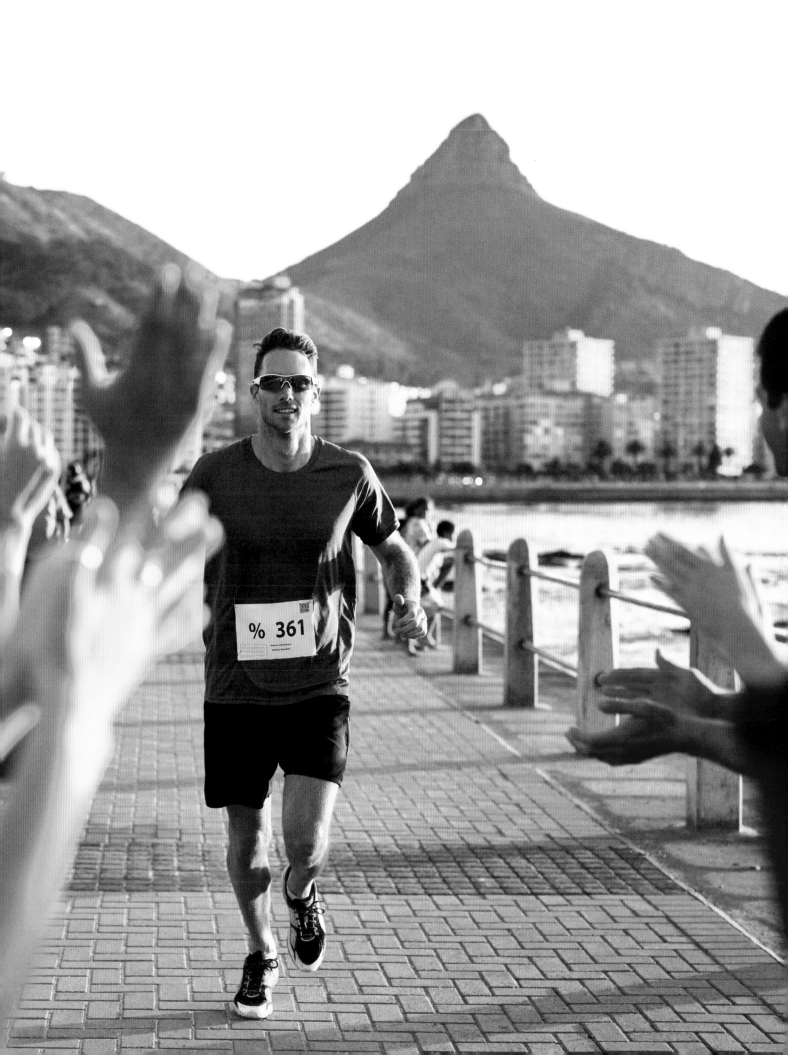

MARATHON TRAINING PLAN FOR BEGINNERS

184

	DAY 1	DAY 2	DAY 3	DAY 4	DAY 5	DAY 6	DAY 7
WEEK 1	Rest, light swim or aerobic cross training session 30 mins Stretch after	Threshold run for 3 x 4 mins 3 mins jog recovery 15 mins warm up / cool down jog	Pilates, yoga or core body conditioning	Continuous hills 3 x 4 mins 15 mins warm up / cool down jog 3 mins recovery between sets	Rest	Rest or 30 mins relaxed run or cross training / swim	Long run - 45 mins easy conversational pace
WEEK 2	Rest, light swim or aerobic cross training session 30 mins Stretch after	Threshold run for 4 x 4 mins 3 mins jog recovery 15 mins warm up / cool down jog	Pilates, yoga or core body conditioning	Continuous hills 3 x 5 mins 15 mins warm up / cool down jog 3 mins recovery between sets	Rest	Rest or 30 mins relaxed run or cross training / swim	Long run - 45-60 mins easy conversational pace
WEEK 3	Rest, light swim or aerobic cross training session 30 mins Stretch after	Threshold run for 3 x 5 mins 3 mins jog recovery 15 mins warm up / cool down jog	Pilates, yoga or core body conditioning	Continuous hills 3 x 5 mins 15 mins warm up / cool down jog 3 mins recovery between sets	Rest	Rest or 30 mins relaxed run or cross training / swim	Long run - 60 mins easy conversational pace
WEEK 4	Rest, light swim or aerobic cross training session 30 mins Stretch after	Threshold run for 4 x 5 mins 3 mins jog recovery 15 mins warm up / cool down jog	Pilates, yoga or core body conditioning	Continuous hills 2 x 7.5 mins 15 mins warm up / cool down jog 3 mins recovery between sets	Rest	Rest or 30 mins relaxed run or cross training / swim	Long run - 75 mins easy conversational pace
WEEK 5	Rest, light swim or aerobic cross training session 30 mins Stretch after	Threshold run for 5 x 5 mins 3 mins jog recovery 15 mins warm up / cool down jog	Pilates, yoga or core body conditioning	Continuous hills 2 x 10 mins 15 mins warm up / cool down jog 3 mins recovery between sets	Rest	Rest or 30 mins relaxed run or cross training / swim	Long run - 90 mins easy conversational pace
WEEK 6	Rest	Recovery run 30 mins	Pilates, yoga or core body conditioning	30 mins run, comprising 5 mins easy 5 mins threshold Repeat x 3	Rest	Rest	Long run 60 mins
WEEK 7	Rest, light swim or aerobic cross training session 30 mins Stretch after	Threshold run for 4 x 6 mins 2 mins jog recovery 15 mins warm up/cool down jog	Pilates, yoga or core body conditioning	Continuous hills 4 x 6 mins 15 mins warm up / cool down jog 3 mins recovery between sets	Rest	Rest or 30 mins relaxed run or cross training / swim	Long run 90 mins with last 30 mins at target marathon pace
WEEK 8	Rest, light swim or aerobic cross training session 30 mins Stretch after	Progression run 10 mins easy 10 mins steady 10 mins at threshold as continuous 30 min run	Pilates, yoga or core body conditioning	Continuous hills 5 x 5 mins effort 3 mins jog recovery between sets	Rest	Rest or 30 mins relaxed run or cross training / swim	Long run - 105 mins easy conversational pace
WEEK 9	Rest, light swim or aerobic cross training session 30 mins Stretch after	Progression run 15 mins easy 15 mins steady 15 mins at threshold as continuous 45 min run	Pilates, yoga or core body conditioning	Continuous hills 4 x 7 mins effort 3 mins jog recovery between sets	Rest	Rest or 45 mins relaxed run or cross training / swim	Long run - 120 mins easy conversational pace
WEEK 10	Rest	Pilates or core conditioning 30 mins recovery run & stretching	Intervals 4 x 5 mins at threshold pace Jog recovery 2-3 mins in between	Rest or 45 mins relaxed cross training / swim	Rest	Recovery run 15 mins plus stretching	Half marathon at target marathon pace
WEEK 11	Rest, light swim or aerobic cross training session 30 mins Stretch after	Pilates or core conditioning 30 mins recovery run & stretching	Cross training & stretching 45 mins	Threshold run for 4 x 6 mins effort 3 mins jog recovery between sets	Rest	Rest or 45 mins relaxed run or cross training / swim	Long run 140 mins with last 40 mins at target marathon pace
WEEK 12	Rest, light swim or aerobic cross training session 30 mins Stretch after	Pilates or core conditioning 30 mins recovery run & stretching	Cross training & stretching 45 mins	Medium run 80 mins with middle 45s min at 3 mins threshold / 3 mins easy	Rest	Rest or 45 mins relaxed run or cross training / swim	Long run 160 mins with 60 mins easy, 60 mins at target marathon pace, 40mins easy
WEEK 13	Rest	Pilates or core conditioning 30 mins recovery run & stretching	Cross training & stretching 45 mins	60 mins including 3 x 10 mins at threshold 3 mins jog recovery between sets	Rest	Rest or 30 mins relaxed run or cross training / swim	Long run 60 mins at easy pace
WEEK 14	Rest	30 mins recovery run	30 mins run incl. 3 x 5 mins easy 5 mins marathon pace	15-20 mins easy jog	Rest	15 mins very easy jog	Marathon

MARATHON TRAINING PLAN FOR IMPROVERS

	DAY 1	DAY 2	DAY 3	DAY 4	DAY 5	DAY 6	DAY 7
WEEK 1	Core conditioning class, yoga or pilates	Recovery run 30 mins	Threshold run for 2 x 10 mins effort with 2 mins recovery between each effort	Cross training or recovery run 30 mins plus core conditioning	Rest	4 x 5 mins continuous hill reps, 2 mins jog recoveries	Long run 90 mins relaxed pace
WEEK 2	Core conditioning class, yoga or pilates	Recovery run 45 mins	5 x 5 mins at threshold with 2 mins jog recoveries	Cross training or recovery run 45 mins plus core conditioning	Rest	2 x 10 mins continuous hill reps, 2 mins jog recoveries	Long run 105 mins relaxed pace
WEEK 3	Core conditioning class, yoga or pilates	Recovery run 30 mins	45 mins incl. 15 mins easy 15 mins steady 15 mins at threshold	Cross training or recovery run 45 mins plus core conditioning	Rest	4 x 6 mins continuous hill reps, 2 mins jog recoveries	Long run 120 mins relaxed pace
WEEK 4	Core conditioning class, yoga or pilates	Recovery run 40 mins	8 x 3 mins; 2 mins jog recovery. Odd numbers at threshold and even numbers at 10K pace	Cross training or recovery run 45 mins plus core conditioning	Rest	5 x 5 mins at threshold pace on a hilly route, with 2 mins jog recoveries	Long run 120-135 mins relaxed pace
WEEK 5	Core conditioning class, yoga or pilates	Recovery run 30 mins	Rest	30 mins run incl. 5 mins easy 5 mins at threshold repeat x 3	Rest	4 x 6 mins of continuous hills with 90 second recoveries	Easy long run 60-75 mins plus core conditioning
WEEK 6	Core conditioning class, yoga or pilates	60 mins with 3 x 10 mins at threshold, 2-3 mins jog recoveries	Intervals 5 x 5 mins at 10K pace 90 second recoveries	30 mins run incl. 5 mins easy 5 mins at threshold repeat x 3	Rest	Recovery run 30-45 mins or cross training	Long run 135 mins with last 45 mins at marathon pace
WEEK 7	Core conditioning class, yoga or pilates	4 x 6 mins of continuous hills 90 second recoveries	Recovery run 30-45 mins or cross training	10 mins at threshold plus 4 x 3 mins at 10K pace plus 10 mins threshold 2 mins recoveries	Rest	45mins run 15mins easy 15mins steady 15mins at threshold plus core conditioning	Long run 150 mins relaxed pace
WEEK 8	Core conditioning class, yoga or pilates	Recovery run 45 mins	Threshold run for 5 x 6 mins effort with 90 second jog recoveries	Recovery run 30 mins plus core conditioning	Rest	Recovery run 45 mins	Long run 90-105 mins with last 45 mins at marathon pace
WEEK 9	Core conditioning class, yoga or pilates	Recovery run 45 mins	6 x 3 mins. Odd numbers at threshold and even at 10K pace; 90 second recoveries	Recovery run 30-45 mins plus easy core conditioning session	Rest	Recovery run 25-30 mins	Half marathon at PB pace. 30 mins slow warm down
WEEK 10	Core conditioning class, yoga or pilates	Recovery run 45 mins or cross training	Recovery run 45 mins or cross training	45 mins run, including 4 x 6 mins at threshold with 2 mins jog recoveries	Rest	Recovery run 45 mins plus core conditioning	Long run 165 mins with last 45 mins at marathon pace
WEEK 11	Core conditioning class, yoga or pilates	Recovery run 45 mins or cross training	RRecovery run 45 mins or cross training	15 mins marathon pace 5 x 3 mins at 10K pace 15 mins marathon pace 2 mins recovery jogs	Rest	Recovery run 45 mins plus core conditioning	Long run 180 mins with last 60 mins at marathon pace
WEEK 12	Core conditioning class, yoga or pilates	Recovery run 30 mins	Recovery run 45 mins	75 mins run, including 3 x 10 mins at threshold	Rest	Recovery run 45 mins plus core conditioning	Long run 120 mins with last hour including 3 x 15 mins at marathon pace
WEEK 13	Core conditioning class, yoga or pilates	Recovery run 30 mins	Recovery run 45 mins or cross training	90 mins run, with middle 60 at 3 mins threshold / 3 mins steady continuous	Rest	5 x 5 mins at threshold with 90 second jog recovery between efforts	Long run 60 mins easy pace, plus core conditioning
WEEK 14	Rest	Recovery run 30 mins plus core conditioning	40 mins incl. 5 mins easy 5 mins at marathon pace repeat x 4	Recovery run 25 mins or cross training	Rest	15 min jog	Marathon

185

26 TIPS FOR YOUR FIRST MARATHON

How to break down the wall, stay injury-free and avoid runner's nipple.

1 TREAT YOURSELF
Buy a good quality pair of running shoes. Go to a good running store where you can get your running style analysed.

2 BACK TO BASICS
Don't be afraid – be excited, because it's a hugely exciting event. Get the basics right. Then, come race day, you can enjoy it.

3 UP THE MILEAGE
One long run a week is essential. Run at an easy, conversational pace, increasing the distance each week. With three weeks to go, aim to cover 20 miles.

4 FORGIVE AND FORGET
There will be the odd day when you have to taxi your kids about or cook dinner or your sofa is just too comfy. That's fine. Don't let training take over your life. It's supposed to be enjoyable.

5 LISTEN TO YOUR BODY
If you want to run but your muscles say otherwise, listen to them. One missed day is better than injury.

6 MIX IT UP
Cross-training is key: core work, weights and plyometrics are great for overall body fitness and strength as they help combat the impact that running has on your body.

7 START LIFTING
Concurrent training – strength and endurance – increases strength and VO_2 max while having a greater effect on fat loss than endurance alone.

8 LESS IS MORE
Your final three weeks of training need to be tapered. Three weeks out, do 75 per cent of your normal mileage, then 50 per cent and finish on 25 per cent with a week to go.

9 IN SYNC
Try and run at the same time of day as the race. When the big day arrives, your mind, body and bladder will be working in harmony.

10 EAT SAFE
Do not eat curry, seafood or anything remotely exotic three days before the race in order to avoid a potentially disastrous stomach upset.

11 PRE-RACE RUN
Go for a very light 15–20-minute run the day before to avoid having the sensation of heavy legs.

12 TRIM YOUR TOENAILS
Make sure you don't have 26.2 miles' worth of snagging nail.

13 DRESS APPROPRIATELY
Don't think about running in a new top. Go for a tried and trusted training-run favourite or have your special charity top worn in beforehand.

14 BE A STAR
Write your name on the back of your top and lap up every cheer, jeer and heckle from your adoring fans.

15 RISE AND SHINE
Get up three or four hours before the race. Eat a balanced breakfast and maybe even have a hot bath to warm your muscles up.

16 START LIGHT
Many runners don't like to run on a full stomach. A light alternative could be something like a cup of simple Greek-style yogurt with some berries or a banana sliced inside and perhaps some nuts.

17 CARB IT UP
Whatever you go for, make sure it's high in carbs. Cereals, toast and porridge are also good options.

18 LUBE UP
Women have sports bras and men need to avoid painful chafing by applying plentiful Vaseline. Keep some plasters for mid-race emergencies.

19 CHILL OUT
Take time to relax and go through your race strategy. Make sure you arrive in plenty of time.

20 KNOW THE COURSE
Think of the marathon as a series of mini-races to get food and drink and have a good idea of when the next station is coming up.

21 PRE-RACE TOILET STOP
Look for a toilet in the start zone. An early break could derail the most promising of starts.

22 START SLOW
Start slow, finish strong. Avoid the urge to storm off like you could come in first.

23 DRINK RESPONSIBLY
Over-hydrating can be a bigger problem than not drinking enough. Drink only when you're thirsty and opt for sports drinks where possible.

24 PLAY GAMES
Count in your head; spot-the-landmark; imagine you're running to save the world; follow a nice figure in front – the simplest distractions can be the most effective.

25 VISUALISE
When you're struggling, imagine how you'll feel that night, curled up in bed, safe in the knowledge that you have achieved your goal.

26 FINISH IN STYLE
As you approach the finish line, make sure you've still got enough energy to raise a smile and stride like you've been leaping the whole way.

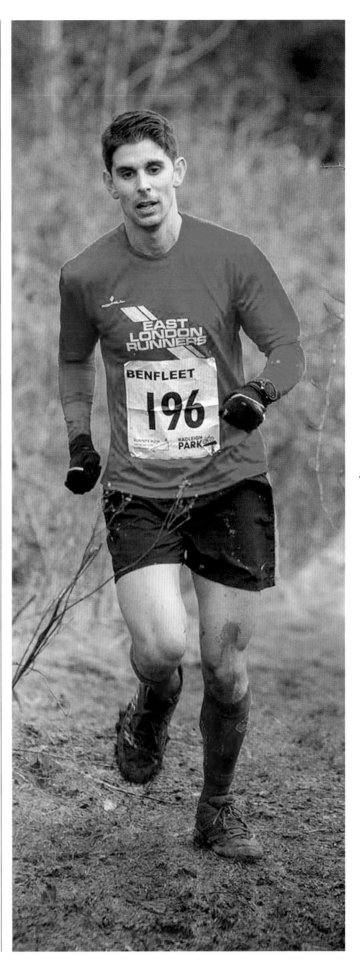

GLOSSARY

Aerobic exercise: brisk exercise that promotes the circulation of oxygen through the blood and is associated with an increased rate of breathing.

Aerobic respiration: the process in which glucose is converted into energy, carbon dioxide and water. During exercise the rate of respiration should increase dramatically.

Altitude training: athletic training that occurs at high altitudes – generally over 5000 feet above sea level. It allows the body to become more efficient in using oxygen, which boosts performance.

Antioxidants: nutrients and proteins in your body that assist in chemical reactions. They are believed to play a role in preventing the development of many chronic diseases.

Arm drive: the movement of the arm while running. An efficient arm drive is vital to setting your rhythm, which in turn dictates your speed.

Basal metabolic rate: the rate at which the body uses energy and burns calories while at rest to maintain vital functions such as breathing.

Biomechanics: the study of the mechanical laws relating to movement of a living organism.

Body composition: the differing percentages of the components of the body, such as muscle, fat, bone etc.

Cadence: the number of steps taken during one minute.

Cadence breathing: the number of breaths taken per step.

Calorie: a unit of measure of the energy released by food as it is digested. One calorie is equivalent to 4.1868 joules.

Carbohydrate: sugars and starches, found in foods such as vegetables, grains, rice, breads and cereals, which are broken down by the body into glucose, the body's principal energy source.

Cardiovascular fitness: the ability of the heart, blood and lungs to supply oxygen-rich blood to muscles, combined with the ability of those muscles to convert oxygen to energy.

Cartilage: a strong tissue that connects joints in the body

Circuit training: a weight training technique in which you move rapidly from exercise to exercise without rest.

Cool down: slow, easy running done after a workout to aid recovery.

Core strength: the strength of the underlying muscles of the torso. These are incredibly important in all forms of athletic endeavor.

Cross training: training in different sports in order to improve general fitness and performance.

Cushioning: the ability of a shoe or surface to minimize the shock of running.

Electrolytes: Vital salts such as sodium, potassium and chloride that are necessary for muscle contraction and maintenance of body fluid levels.

Endurance: the ability to run long distances.

Energy gels: carbohydrate gels that provide energy for both active running and to promote recovery.

Fartlek: a workout that includes faster running mixed with slower running.

Fat: the most concentrated source of food energy, supplying nine calories per gram. Stored fat provides about half the energy for low-intensity exercise.

Fell running: running or racing off-road, particularly over hills where the gradient of running greatly increases the difficulty.

Flexibility training: a workout that improves the range of flexibility; the range of motion of your joints.

Foam rolling: a self-myofascial release technique particularly useful for massaging tight muscles and knots after training.

Foot strike: in the running stride, the moment of contact between the runner's foot and the ground.

Glucose: the main type of sugar in blood, and the body's preferred source of energy

Glutes: the gluteal muscles of the buttocks.

Glycemic index: a figure representing the relative ability of a carbohydrate food to increase the level of glucose in the blood.

Glycogen stores: the form in which carbohydrates are stored in the body, primarily in muscles and the liver.

GPS: stands for Global Positioning System, and is a radio navigation that enables runners to identify where they are and track the speed and distance run.

Green exercise: physical exercise undertaken outdoors in green, natural areas.

Half marathon: a race of 13.1 miles, or 21.1 kilometers.
Hill reps: a workout that involves running hard up a hill. Useful both for endurance and for strength training in the major running muscles.
Hydration: the process by which water in ingested and absorbed into the body. A healthy level of hydration is key for any athletic exercise.
Hyponatraemia: a dangerously low sodium level in the blood which can be caused by drinking too much water.

Ice bath: a freezing-cold post-training bath which helps recovery by constricting blood vessels, reducing swelling and removing waste products.
Interval sessions: a workout that involves running a set distance repeatedly with a recovery jog in between.

Jogging: the activity of running at a steady, reasonably slow pace. A jogging pace should be one that you can maintain over long distances.
Junk Miles: runs used to reach a weekly or monthly mileage goal, rather than for a specific training purpose.

Lactic acid: a waste by-product of the breakdown of glucose that forms in the muscles. Associated with muscle fatigue and cramp.
Ligaments: short bands of tough, flexible fibrous tissue connecting bones or cartilage at a joint.
Lunges: useful cross-training exercise where one leg is positioned forward with knee bent and foot flat.
Marathon: a race of 26.2 miles, or 42.2 kilometers.

Nutrition: the process of providing the food the body needs for health and growth.
Overtraining: condition when a runner trains too much, leading to fatigue and injury.

Pace: measurement of the speed of running.
Peak: scheduling training so that the best performance is achieved at a race or event.
Physiotherapy: the treatment of injury or fatigue by physical methods such as massage, heat treatment and exercise.
Pilates: a system of exercises designed to improve physical strength, flexibility and posture.
Pronation: the natural, inward roll of the foot that occurs when the heel strikes the ground. Correct pronation is important for a sustainable running style.
Protein: nutrient required for tissue growth and repair.

Recovery time: the amount of time taken to return to normal physical fitness.
Repetitions: each individual exercise in a longer workout. Often known as reps.

Split: the time taken to run certain distances (often a mile) during a longer run.
Sports massage: specially-designed massages that promote flexibility reduce fatigue, improve endurance and help prevent injury.

Sprint: a short-distance run at full speed.
Strength training: physical exercise specializing in the use of resistance to induce muscular contraction which builds the strength and endurance of muscles.

Tapering: a period of semi-rest before a big competition, usually a week or two before a big race.
Tempo running: a type of running designed to boost speed and endurance, during which the aim is to run at about 75 per cent of maximum effort.
Tendons: a flexible but inelastic cord of strong fibrous collagen tissue attaching a muscle to a bone.
Threshold running: a run carried out at an intensity just below the point where your body would not be able to remove the acid waste build-up in the muscles.
Trail running: a form of running which takes place away from roads and tracks; generally over hiking trails, or on mountainous terrain.

Ultra-marathon: a race that is longer than a marathon in distance.

VO2 max: the maximum amount of oxygen that can be utilized by the body.

Wall: a state of exhaustion when your body runs out of glycogen or energy. Often at the 20-mile point in a marathon.

Yoga: a Hindu spiritual discipline, widely practiced for health and relaxation.

INDEX

191

PICTURE CREDITS

The publishers would like to thank the following sources for their kind permission to reproduce the pictures in this book.

Emily Clarke: 29TL, 29TR, 29BR, 30-31C, 30TR, 30B, 51, 158L, 158R

Getty Images: /Janie Airey/Photodisc: 77; /Fuse/Corbis: 40; /Ryan McVay/ DigitalVision: 85TR; /Medioimages/Photodisc: 136BR

iStockphoto: 3, 4-5, 6-7, 8, 9, 10-11, 12, 13, 14, 15, 17, 18, 20, 21, 22, 23, 24, 25, 27, 28TR, 28L, 28BR, 30C, 31T, 33, 34-35, 36, 37, 41, 43, 45, 46, 47, 53, 55, 56L, 56R, 57TR, 57BR, 59, 60, 61, 62, 63, 71, 72, 73, 75, 76, 79, 81, 83, 84, 85BL, 85BR, 86, 87, 88-89, 91L, 91R, 92, 93, 96, 97, 118BL, 118TR, 119, 120T, 120B, 121, 123, 124, 125, 126-127, 128, 129, 130, 131, 133, 134, 135, 136BC, 137, 138, 139, 140TR, 140C, 140BC, 140BR, 141TL, 141TR, 141C, 141BL, 141BC, 142T, 142R, 142B, 143TL, 143TR, 143BL, 143BR, 144-145, 147, 148, 149, 150, 151, 153BR, 157, 159L, 161L, 163, 165, 167, 169, 170-171, 175, 178, 179, 183

Peter Liddiard: 94-95, 106-107, 108-109, 110-111, 112, 113T, 113B, 114, 115

Antonio Romero: 187

Shutterstock: 3

Thinkstock: 38, 39, 90

Wild Bunch Media Limited: 29BL, 31B, 99L, 99R, 102-103, 153L, 155, 159R, 160L, 160TR, 160BR, 161R, 164, 166; /Eddie MacDonald: 19, 57L, 64-65, 66-67, 70, 104-105, 116-117, 152

Ellie Wilkinson: 42

Every effort has been made to acknowledge correctly and contact the source and/or copyright holder of each picture and Carlton Books Limited apologises for any unintentional errors or omissions that will be corrected in future editions of this book.